# FITNESS SUTRA

## EXERCISES WITH RESISTANCE LOOP BANDS

### (REVISED 2ND EDITION)

40+ Exercises to Strengthen your Muscles

& Sculpt your Body at Home

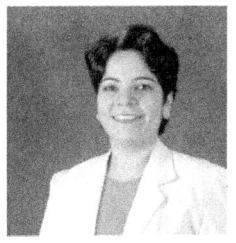

Dr. Monika Chopra
www.fitness-sutra.com

## Dr. Monika Chopra's Fitness Sutra

Copyright © Dr. Monika Chopra, 2019. All rights reserved.

Published by FitSutra Wellness Pvt Ltd,
33, Prachi Residency, Baner Rd., Pune-411045, India

ISBN-13: 978-1-0779-5488-5

No part of this book may be reproduced, transmitted, or utilized in any form or by any means, electronic or mechanical including photocopying or recording or by any information storage and retrieval system, without written permission from the author.

Although I am a Physiotherapist (PT, for those of you in the USA) and a trained Yoga teacher, my suggestions through this book do not establish a doctor-patient relationship between us. This book is not intended to be a substitute for the medical advice of physicians. You should regularly consult a physician in matters relating to your health particularly with respect to any symptoms that may require diagnosis or medical attention. I advise you to take full responsibility of your safety and be aware of your physical limits. Before practising the exercises described in this book, be sure that your equipment is well maintained. Do not take risks beyond your level of flexibility, aptitude, strength, and comfort level.

This is a work of nonfiction. No names have been changed, no characters invented and no events fabricated. The information provided within this Book is for general informational purposes only. While I have tried to keep the information up-to-date and correct, there are no representations or warranties, expressed or implied, about the completeness, accuracy, reliability, suitability or availability with respect to the information, products, services, or related graphics contained in this book for any purpose. Any use of this information is at the reader's own responsibility. I do not assume and hereby disclaim any liability to any party for any loss, damage, or disruption caused by errors or omissions, whether such errors or omissions result from negligence, accident, or any other cause.

Exercises with Resistance Loop Bands (2nd Edition)

# CONTENTS

| | | |
|---|---|---|
| 1 | An Introduction to Resistance Loop Bands | 1 |
| 2 | Resistance Loop Band Basics | 5 |
| 3 | Warm-Up Exercises | 13 |
| 4 | Upper Body Exercises | 21 |
| | Front Triceps Extension | 22 |
| | Rear Triceps Extension | 24 |
| | Horizontal Arm Extension | 26 |
| | Vertical Arm Extension | 28 |
| | Rear Arm Extension | 30 |
| | Bicep Curl | 32 |
| | Internal Rotation | 34 |
| | External Rotation | 36 |
| | Hand Scrunches | 38 |
| | Bear Crawls | 40 |
| | Lateral Arm Raise (Rotator Cuff) | 42 |
| | Seated Concentration Curl | 44 |
| | Wrist Curl | 46 |

| | |
|---|---|
| **5 Lower Body Exercises** | **49** |
| Bridge Thrust | 50 |
| One Leg Hip Thrust | 52 |
| Side Step Squats | 54 |
| Lying Hip Abduction | 56 |
| Lying Leg Raise | 58 |
| Standing Hip Abduction | 60 |
| Band Squats | 62 |
| Leg Extension | 64 |
| Clam Shell | 66 |
| Thigh Thrust | 68 |
| Lateral Walk | 70 |
| Standing Hip Flexion | 72 |
| Single Leg Loop Bridge | 74 |
| Backwards Leg Swing | 76 |
| Standing Hip Adduction | 78 |
| Standing Hip Extension | 80 |
| Seated Leg Extension | 82 |
| Seated Hip Abduction | 84 |
| Ankle Internal Rotation | 86 |

Exercises with Resistance Loop Bands (2nd Edition)

|  |  |  |
|---|---|---|
|  | Supinated Clamshell | 88 |
| 6 | Chest & Back Exercises | 89 |
|  | Lateral Push Up | 90 |
|  | Lateral Pull Down | 92 |
|  | Press to Pull | 94 |
|  | Shoulder Retraction | 96 |
|  | Single Arm Rowing | 98 |
| 7 | Abdominal Exercises | 101 |
|  | Oblique Overhead Extension | 102 |
|  | Bicycles | 104 |
|  | Abdominal Crunch with Rotations | 106 |
|  | Reverse Crunch | 108 |
| 8 | Cool-Down Exercises | 110 |
| 9 | Importance of Diet | 119 |
| 10 | Training Regimes | 122 |
| 11 | Bonus | 127 |

Dr. Monika Chopra's Fitness Sutra

# CHAPTER 1

An Introduction to Resistance Loop Bands

## Dr. Monika Chopra's Fitness Sutra

Resistance loop band training is a simple and effective way of doing your resistance exercise to increase muscle tone, muscle strength, burn fat or simply increase body flexibility. It is very cost effective and can be used on the go. It is safe for the beginners and at the same time can be made very challenging for experienced users.

In this book, through step by step instructions, I will guide you to the safe and effective methods of using resistance loop bands. Emphasis will be laid on the correct grasping of the band, proper start position and correct movement of the particular body part for the desired results.

Finally I will guide you to beginners and advanced training regimes which will help you to set desired goals.

*What are resistance loop bands and how are they more useful than free weights or resistance bands?*

Resistance loop bands are the resistance bands that come in the form of one continuous loop. With the loop you can perform the resistance exercises better than the conventional resistance band unit by targeting the workout of a specific muscle. One unambiguous advantage of resistance loop band is that, as you stretch the loop band the resistance level increases thus providing a progressive increase in the muscle stress, which cannot occur with conventional free weights.

With resistance loop band you can do whole range of exercises involving all muscles of your body in various

# Exercises with Resistance Loop Bands (2nd Edition)

ways. These can also be used in conjunction with conventional exercises, thus making them more challenging or more achievable.

## *Why resistance loop bands?*

Resistance loop bands have been used since ages for rehabilitation purpose. They provide a safe and effective method to strengthen up the muscles, ligaments, tendons and joints. Off late their popularity have increased amongst fitness enthusiasts because of ease and effectiveness of their usage. With just your body and your band you're not too far from the gym.

Here are some of the benefits of resistance loop band training.

1. They are effective in strength training exercises.
2. They can be used anywhere – home, office and outdoors.
3. They are portable and storable. They take up little space and are lighter than the free weights.
4. They are extremely cost effective alternative to purchasing bulky gym equipment or taking expensive gym memberships.
5. Resistance loop bands are more versatile as they don't work against force of gravity. They are able to provide freer range of motion than barbells or dumbbells.
6. With resistance loop bands muscles can work both through concentric and eccentric parts of an exercise.

## *Resistance loop band strength levels*

Resistance loop bands have a restoring force that comes in action when the loop is stretched. This restoring force or resistance is linear in nature and varies with the stretch i.e. the more the band is stretched the more is the resistance force. This linear variable resistance helps to engage the fast twitch muscle fibre effectively, thus strengthening them better. Resistance loop band training when combined with free weights provide isotonic workout with linear resistance training which provides better body toning and strengthening.

The resistance level of most band systems follow a colour coded system based on the thickness of the band. The thicker the band, the more is the resistance level. Unfortunately, the colour scheme across brands is not standard and varies with the manufacturer.

Resistance levels and colour codes of a typical brand are given below for reference. You should refer to the band resistance chart of your own loop bands.

| Band Colour | Resistance Levels |
| --- | --- |
| Yellow | Extra Light |
| Green | Light |
| Red | Medium |
| Blue | Heavy |
| Black | Extra Heavy |

# CHAPTER 2

## Resistance Loop Band Basics

## Grips

### Up Grip

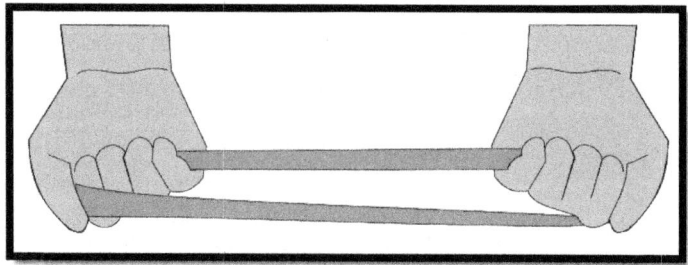

In up grip the band is held in the palms facing up, with fingers enclosing the band fully. It is mainly used in exercises where you have to curl or row the band towards your body, such as biceps curls.

### Down Grip

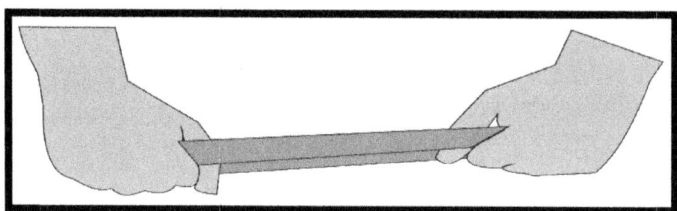

In down grip the band is held in the palms facing down, with fingers enclosing the band fully. It is mainly used for exercises which involve pushing the band away from your body (with the aid of a fixed anchor) or those that have you pulling the resistance toward you.

## Hammer Grip

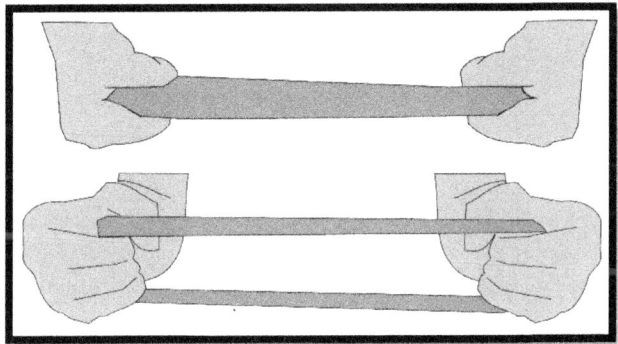

In hammer grip you hold the band in your fist, with both palms facing each other.

## Open Hand Grip

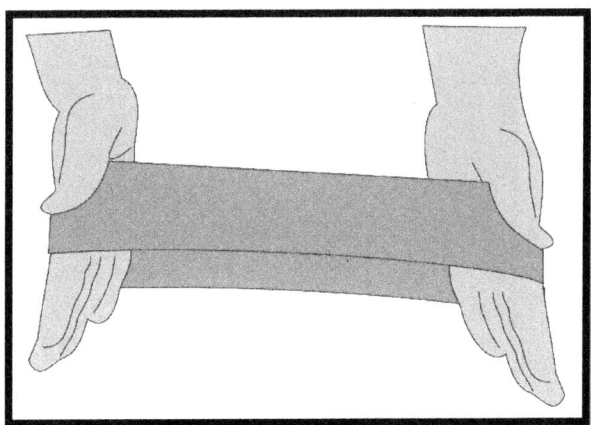

In open hand grip the band is wrapped around the open hands. It is normally used in pulling the band away from the body.

## Wrist Alignment

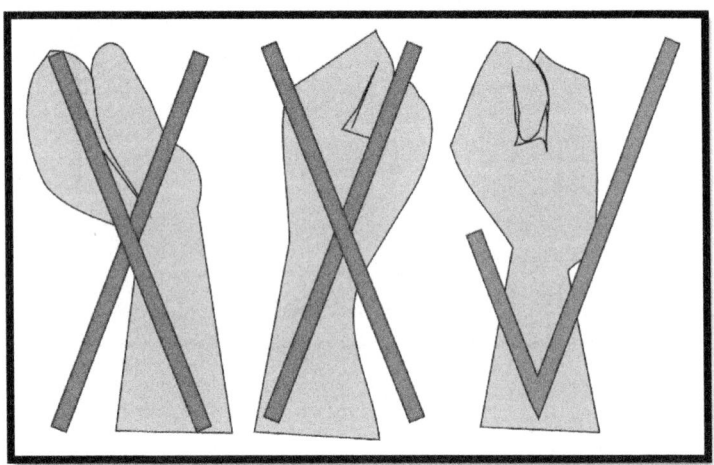

The band should be held in hand with wrist in neutral position i.e. hand should be in line with the forearm (neither extended nor flexed).

## Ready Position

Stand tall with your feet hip width distance apart, shoulders and hips squared (facing forward), gluteal (hip) muscles contracted, knees soft with thigh muscles contracted, arms by the side of your body and looking straight forward.

# Exercises with Resistance Loop Bands (2nd Edition)

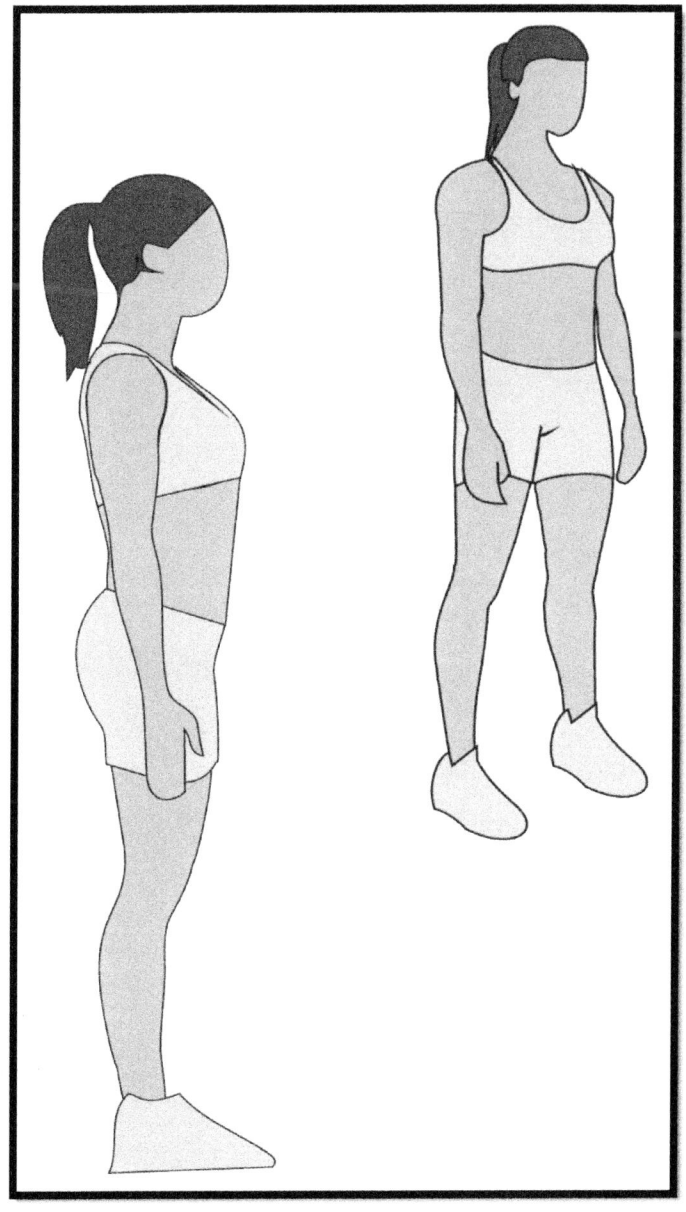

Dr. Monika Chopra's Fitness Sutra

How to use the Band

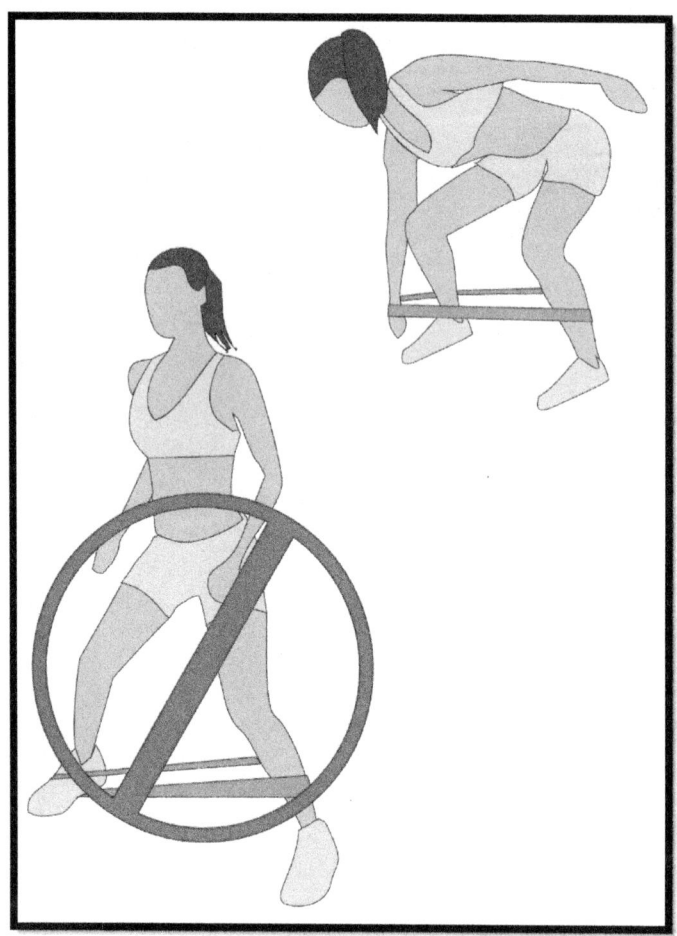

- Use the band only as directed.
- Never stretch the band in the direction of face or other sensitive parts of the body.

# Exercises with Resistance Loop Bands (2nd Edition)

- Never stretch the band more than 2½ times its resting length.
- If desired resistance is not achieved, when using according to directions, switch to a band that provides desired resistance.
- Inspect for possible wear and tear before use. Discontinue use if torn.
- Perform your workout on carpeted surface, wood floors or grass.
- Do not use on abrasive surface. Abrasive surface like cement or asphalt can damage the band.
- Keep away from children.
- You should also check the specific instructions that came with your set of bands. Sometimes the materials used in the manufacturing may have some peculiar properties.

Make sure that when you put a resistance loop band around your ankles, you put it around your feet with both hands. When you take it off, make sure you take it off with both hands. Do not kick them off or try to take them off with your shoes. Doing so can damage the band.

Dr. Monika Chopra's Fitness Sutra

# Bonus

I hope you are finding this book useful and are ready to start with the exercises.

I have also created easy to use quick reference charts of the regimes (beginners / advanced), suggested in the last chapter of this book. These can be downloaded as ready printable files from

https://www.fitness-sutra.com/go?id=121070

 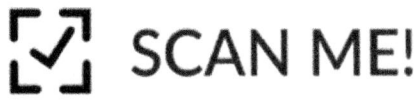

You can also subscribe to my mailing list to get more tips & motivation to do these exercises. To top it all, you would get a chance to download a FREE copy of this book when I come out with the next revision.

# CHAPTER 3

## Warm-Up Exercises

To stay safe and prepare your body for exercises you should always do some warm ups before the resistance exercises. The warm up exercises help to increase the temperature and loosen the muscles before the heavy body muscle work. Warm ups improve the body performance and prevent injuries. These exercises should be dynamic exercises like skipping, jogging at a place, chest expansion & rotations. About 5 minutes' warm ups are enough to make your cardiovascular system ready.

The following warm up exercises are good to prepare your body for intense workout (Do 10 repetitions per exercise).

1. <u>Neck Rotations:</u>

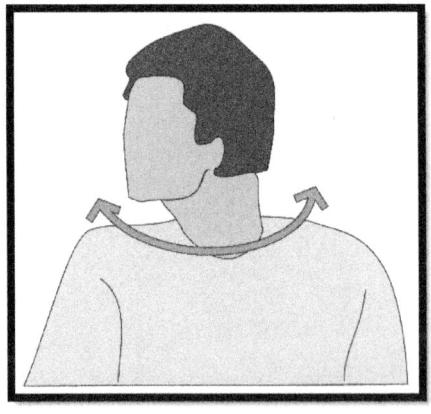

Stand tall with your chin parallel to the ground. Exhale and take your chin to the chest. Inhale, rotate your neck and take your chin towards the left shoulder (look over your left shoulder). Exhale and get your chin back to the chest position. Inhale, rotate your neck and take your chin to the right shoulder (look over your right shoulder). Get your chin back to the chest position as you exhale. Move your chin up to the start position as you inhale. Repeat 3 times.

Exercises with Resistance Loop Bands (2nd Edition)

2. Shoulder Backward Rotations:

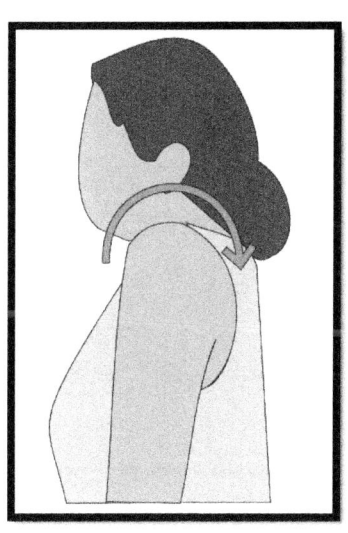

Stand tall with chin parallel to the floor and shoulders facing forward. Take your shoulders forward. Start rotating the shoulders taking them up and behind. Get your shoulder-blades together as you move the shoulders behind. Get shoulders back to the start position. Repeat this sequence 10 times.

3. Shoulder Forward Rotations:

Stand tall with chin parallel to the floor and shoulders facing forward. Take your shoulders behind, getting your shoulder blades together. Continue rotating the shoulders taking them up and forwards. Get shoulders back to the start position. Repeat this sequence 10 times.

4. <u>Chest Expansions:</u>

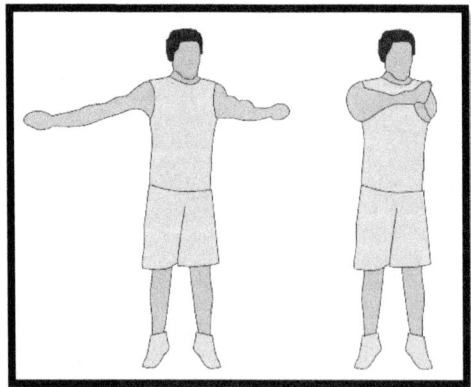

Stand tall with chin parallel to the floor and shoulders facing forward. Raise your arms to the shoulder level and take them back opening the chest. Repeat 10 times.

5. <u>Torso Rotations:</u>

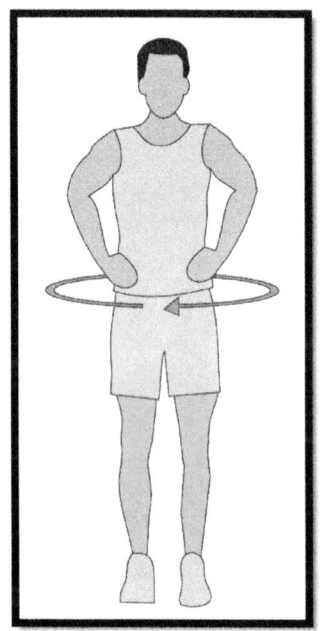

Stand tall with feet hip width distance apart. Place your hands on the waist and rotate your trunk clockwise. Repeat 10 times. Then rotate your trunk anti-clockwise. Repeat 10 times.

Exercises with Resistance Loop Bands (2nd Edition)

6.     Arm Rotations:

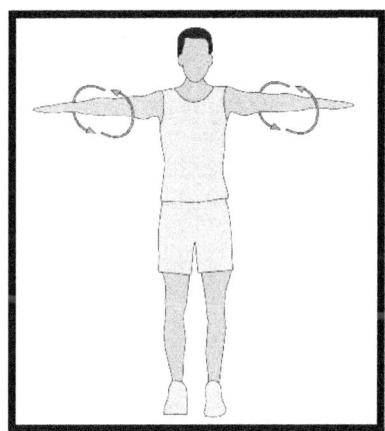

Stand tall with your feet hip width distance apart. Raise your arms to the side at shoulder level. Make circles with your arms moving them clockwise and anti-clockwise (10 times in each direction).

7.     Side Arm Raises:

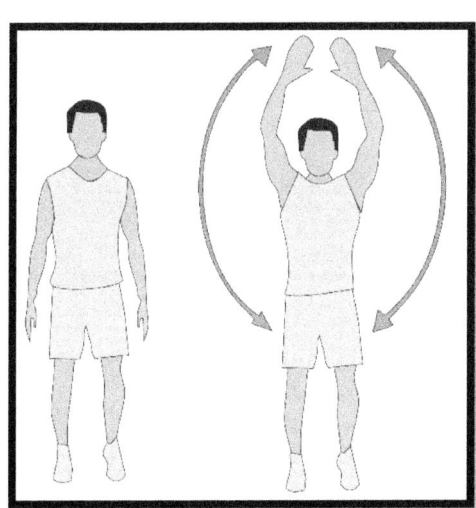

Stand tall with your feet hip width distance apart. Raise your both arms sideways up 10 times.

Dr. Monika Chopra's Fitness Sutra

8.     <u>Hip Rotation</u>

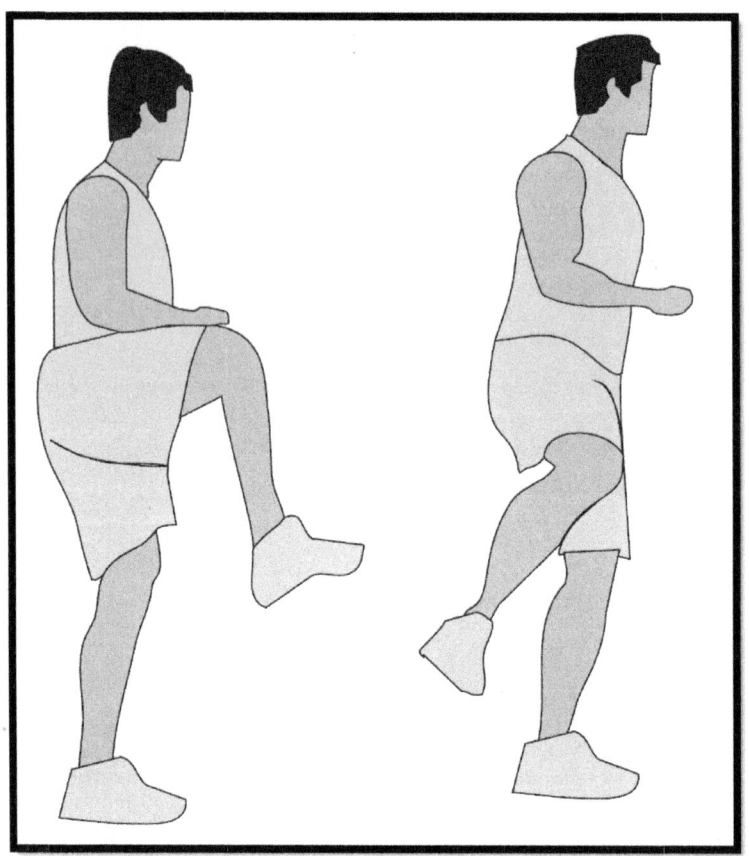

Lift your right leg and balance your body on the left foot. Rotate your leg at the hips in clockwise direction 10 times. Next rotate it in reverse direction 10 times. Repeat with the other leg.

Exercises with Resistance Loop Bands (2nd Edition)

9. Jog on Spot

Jog on the spot. Try to lift your legs high enough to make your thighs parallel to the ground. Do 20 jogs of each foot.

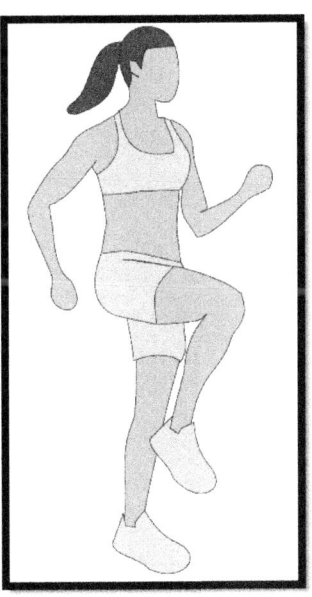

10. Side to Side Hop

Balance yourself on one foot with the other leg raised high. Hop on the raised leg side, bringing that one down and raising the other leg up simultaneously. Repeat this 20 times.

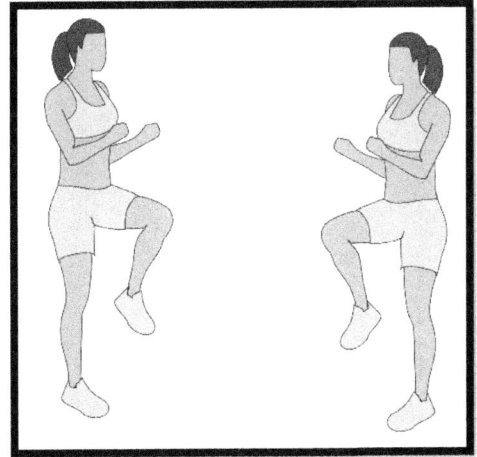

<u>Warm-up Sets:</u> Every exercise you want to perform should begin with a warm up set. Warm up set includes all the exercises you are going to do, with little or no resistance for 10-15 repetitions with slower than normal tempo. So if you are working with a red band, you should do the warm-up with a green band.

# CHAPTER 4

## Upper Body Exercises

Dr. Monika Chopra's Fitness Sutra

## Front Triceps Extension

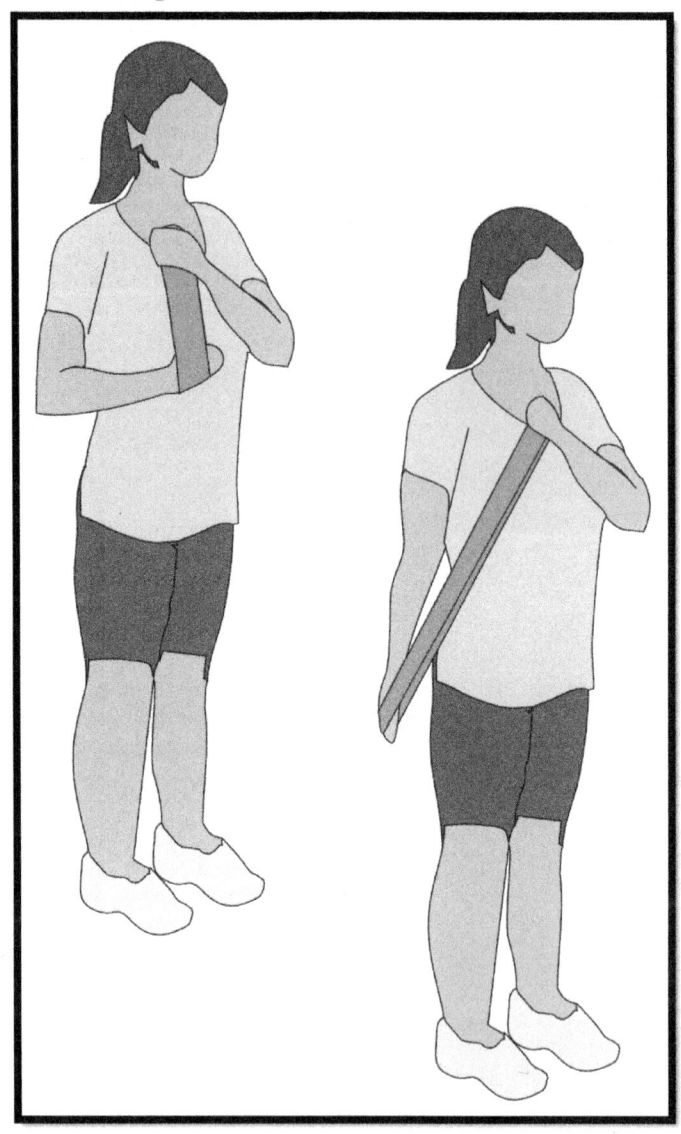

# Exercises with Resistance Loop Bands (2nd Edition)

*Effect:* This exercise mainly works on strengthening of the triceps muscles.

*Difficulty Level:* Beginner

*Start Position:* Stand tall with feet shoulder width apart. Hold one end of the band in hammer grip in left hand and brace it against your left collar bone. Hold the other end of the band in your right hand against your chest with open hand grip.

*Steps:*

1. Keeping your right elbow tucked in by the side of your trunk, push your right arm to full extension.
2. Hold the stretched position for 5 counts and then release the stretch slowly returning the arm to the start position.
3. Do required number of repetitions.
4. Repeat on the left side.

*Fine Tips:*

1. Make sure that the left hand stays in a braced position at your chest as you take the right hand down and vice versa.
2. The movement should be slow and controlled.

## Rear Triceps Extension

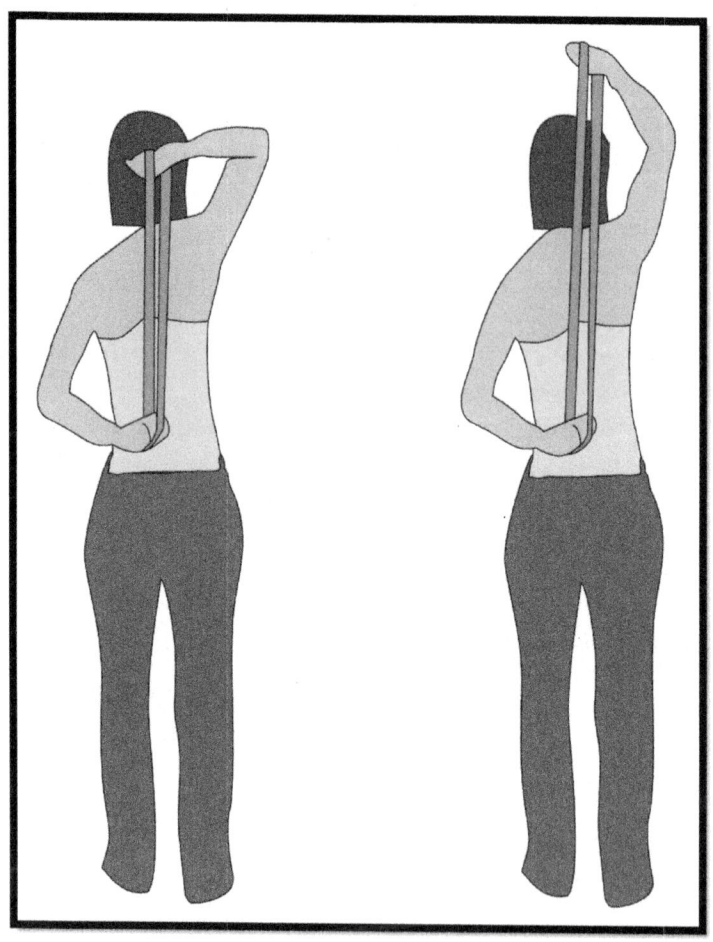

# Exercises with Resistance Loop Bands (2nd Edition)

*Effect:* This exercise works on mainly strengthening of the triceps muscles.

*Difficulty Level:* Advanced

*Start Position:* Stand tall with your feet shoulder width apart. Raise right elbow to forehead level and hold one end of the resistance loop in right hand with up grip. Drop the other end of the resistance loop behind your back and hold it with the left hand (hand facing out).

*Steps:*

1. Keeping the left hand stable extend the right arm, pulling the band up.
2. Hold the stretched position for 5 counts and then release the stretch and bring it back to the start position.
3. Do required number of repetitions.
4. Repeat on the other side.

*Fine Tips:*

1. The movement should be slow and controlled.
2. Do not lock your elbow in full extension position.

Dr. Monika Chopra's Fitness Sutra

# Horizontal Arm Extension

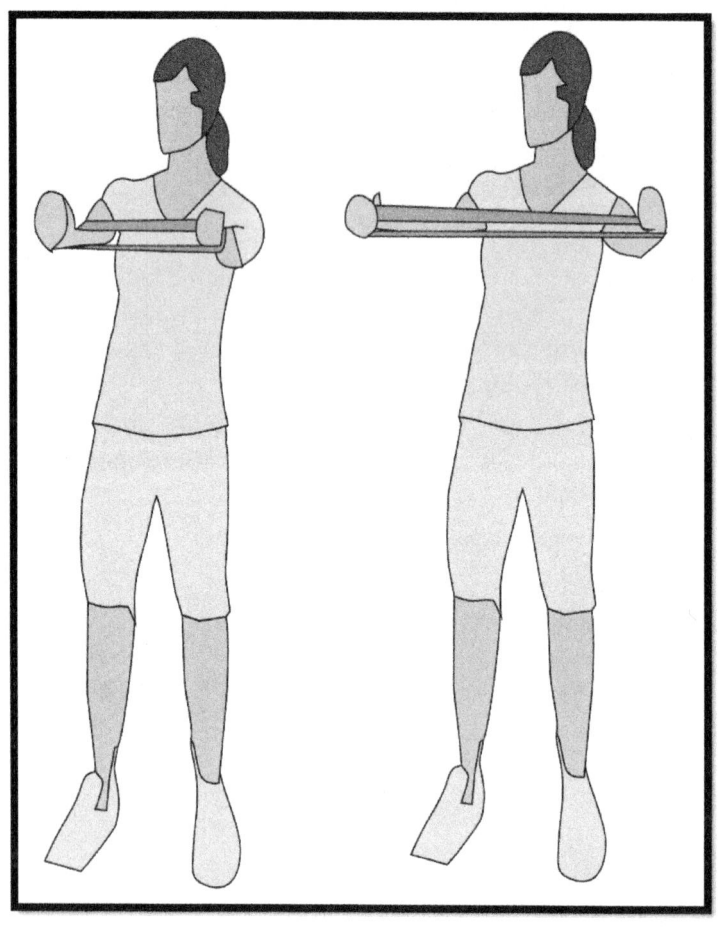

# Exercises with Resistance Loop Bands (2$^{nd}$ Edition)

*Effect:* This exercise works on strengthening of back arm (abductors) and upper back muscles

*Difficulty Level:* Beginner

*Start Position:* Stand tall with back straight and feet shoulder width apart. Place the resistance band around your wrists and extend your arms in front of you at shoulder level, hands shoulder width apart.

*Steps:*

1. Keeping arms slightly bent at elbows, pull the band apart by applying outward pressure to your forearms. Move the arms horizontally maintaining them at shoulder level.
2. Hold the stretched position for 5 counts.
3. Release the stretch and return to the start position.
4. Do required number of repetitions.

*Fine Tips:*

1. The movement should be slow and controlled.
2. Do not lock the elbow at any time during the movement.

## Dr. Monika Chopra's Fitness Sutra

## Vertical Arm Extension

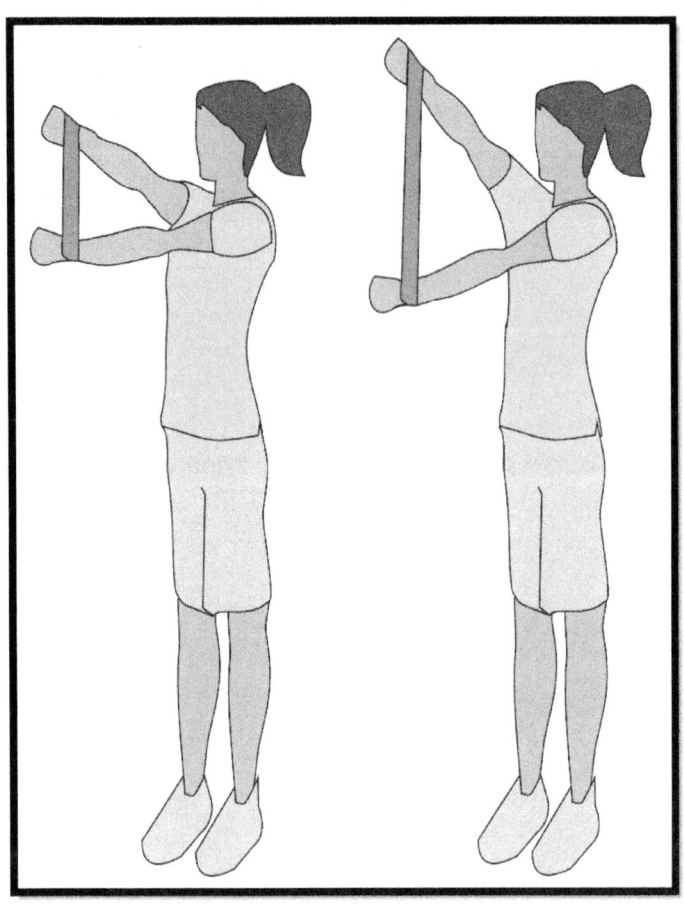

# Exercises with Resistance Loop Bands (2nd Edition)

*Effect:* This exercise helps in strengthening arm extensor and flexor muscles.

*Difficulty Level:* Beginner

*Start Position:* Stand tall with feet shoulder width apart, arms stretched in front of you with left arm at shoulder level and right arm above it and the band around the forearm.

*Steps:*

1. Keeping your arms slightly bent at elbows, pull the band apart by applying upward pressure to right forearm and downward pressure to left forearm. The arms move in the vertical plane. Hold the stretched position for 5 counts.
2. Return to the start position.
3. Switch the arms and repeat.
4. Do required number of repetitions.

*Fine Tips:*

1. The movement should be slow and controlled.
2. Do not lock your elbows anytime during the movement.

## Rear Arm Extension

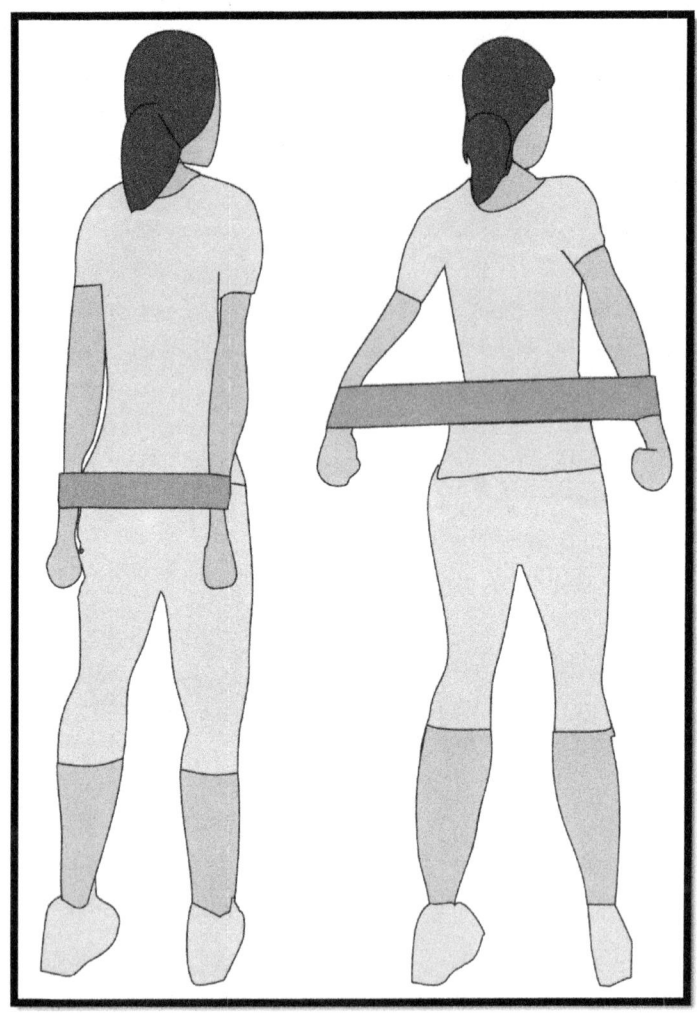

# Exercises with Resistance Loop Bands (2nd Edition)

*Effect:* This exercise works mainly on the strengthening of arms and shoulders abductor muscles in retracted position.

*Difficulty Level:* Advanced

*Start Position:* Stand tall with back straight and feet shoulder width apart. Place the resistance band around your wrists and hold your arm behind you.

*Steps:*

1. Keeping your arms slightly bent, pull the band apart by applying outward pressure to your forearms. Your arms move in horizontal plane.
2. Hold the stretched position for 5 counts.
3. Return to the start position.
4. Repeat required number of times.

*Fine Tips:*

1. The movement should be slow and controlled.
2. Do not lock your elbows throughout the movement.

## Bicep Curl

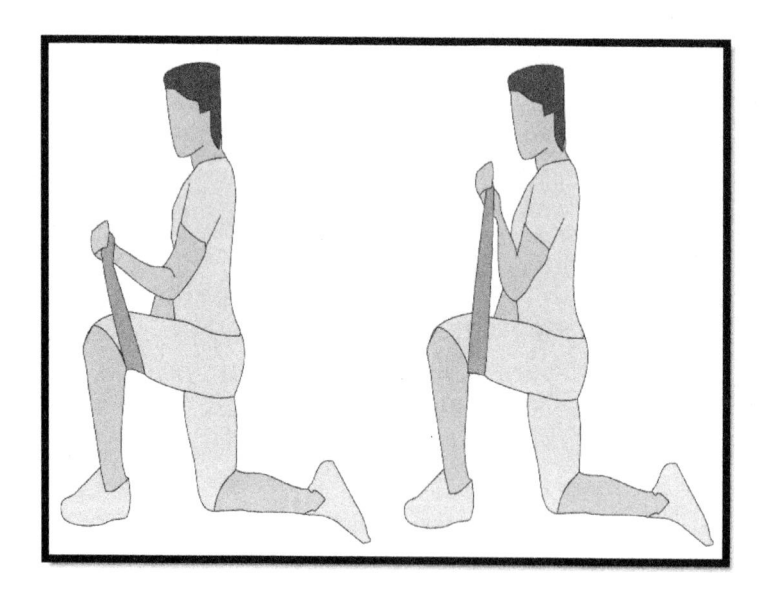

# Exercises with Resistance Loop Bands (2nd Edition)

*Effect:* This exercise works on strengthening of biceps muscles.

*Difficulty Level:* Beginner

*Start Position:* Do a lunge with right knee touching the ground. Loop the resistance band around your left knee, and hold the other end in your left hand with up grip.

*Steps:*

1. Keeping your back tall and abdomen tucked in, curl the arm at elbow, pulling the band up.
2. Squeeze the biceps tightly in the fully contracted position. Hold for 5 counts.
3. Slowly lower to the start position.
4. Repeat required number of times.
5. Repeat on the other side.

*Fine Tips:*

1. Keep your arm tucked by the side of your trunk throughout the movement.
2. The movement should be slow and controlled.

## Internal Rotation

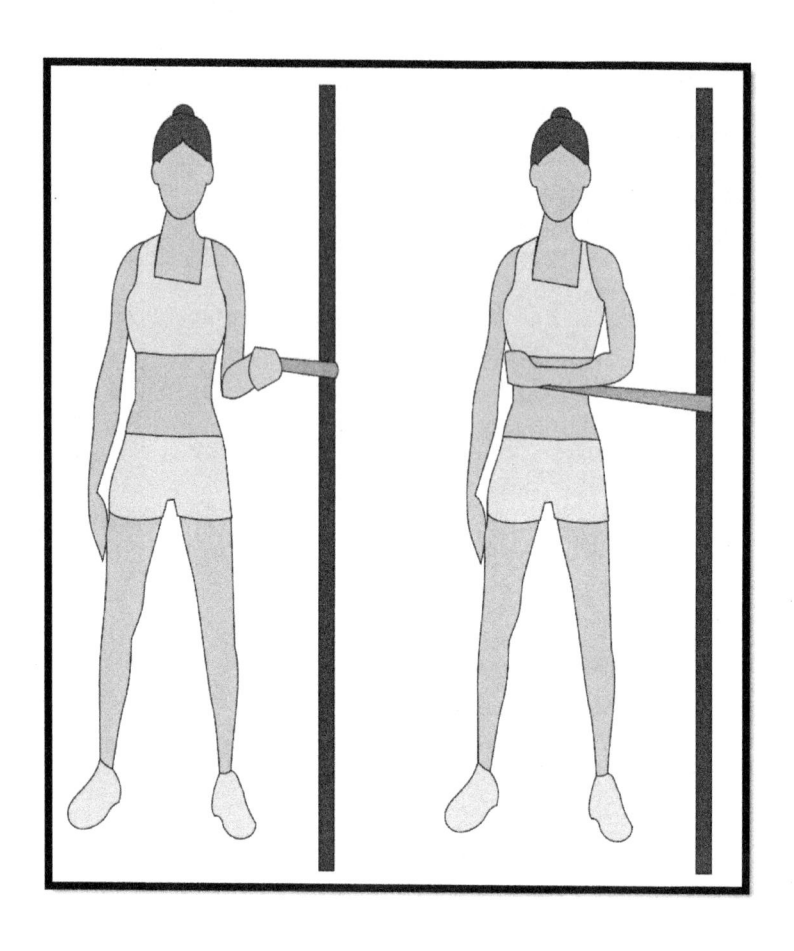

# Exercises with Resistance Loop Bands (2nd Edition)

*Effect:* This exercise works on strengthening of the arm and shoulder internal rotator muscles

*Difficulty Level:* Beginner

*Start Position:* Stand tall, abdomen tucked in, gluteus tight and feet hip width distance apart. Loop the resistance band through a support (like the window rail). Hold the other end of the band in hammer grip, keeping arm tucked by side of the trunk and forearm at 90 degrees to the upper arm, parallel to the floor.

*Steps:*

1. Pull the band inward, taking forearm horizontally to the abdomen.
2. Hold the stretched position for 5 counts and then slowly release bringing forearm back to the start position.
3. Repeat required number of times.
4. Repeat with the other arm.

*Fine Tips:*

1. The movement should be slow and controlled.
2. Keep your arm tucked by the side of the trunk throughout the movement.

# Dr. Monika Chopra's Fitness Sutra

## External Rotation

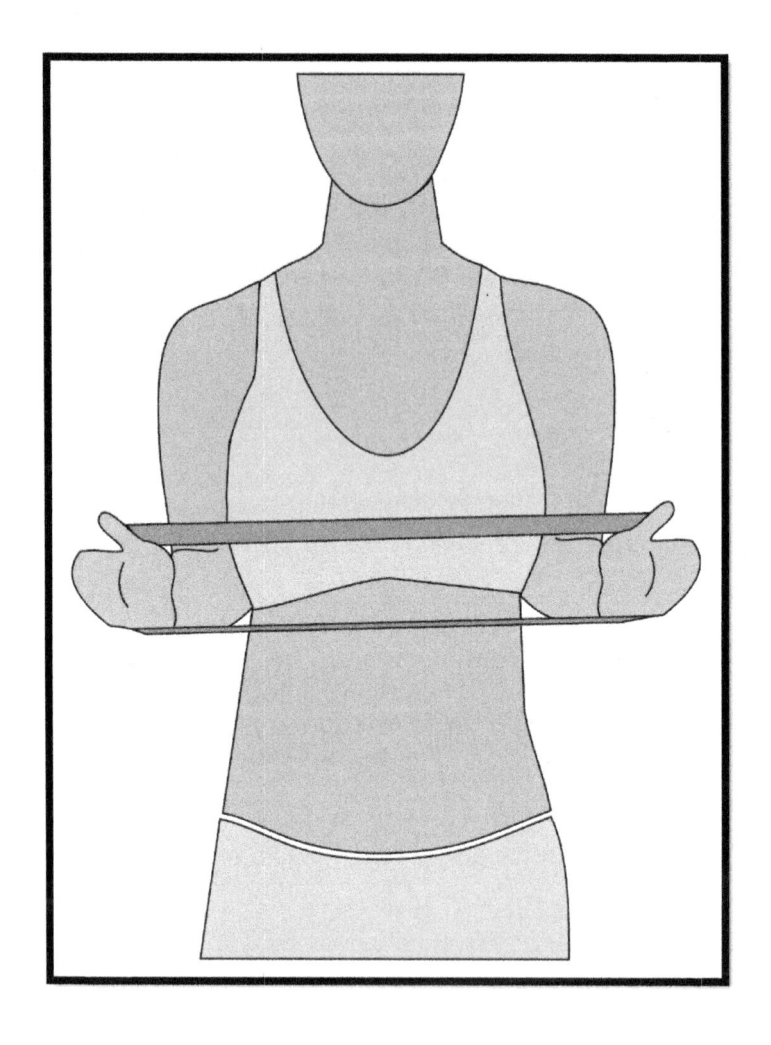

*Effect:* This exercise works on strengthening of arms and shoulders external rotator muscles.

*Difficulty Level:* Beginner

*Start Position:* Stand tall, with back straight, abdomen tucked in and feet hip width distance apart. Hold the resistance loop in open hand grip with both hands, with elbows tucked by side of the trunk and forearms at 90 degrees to the arm, parallel to the floor.

*Steps:*

1. Pull the band horizontally outwards, moving the hands apart, keeping your elbows tucked by the side of the trunk.
2. Hold the stretched position for 5 counts and release.
3. Release the stretch and return your arms to the start position.
4. Repeat required number of times.

*Fine Tips:*

1. Keep your elbows tucked by the side of your trunk throughout the movement.
2. The movement should be slow and controlled.

# Dr. Monika Chopra's Fitness Sutra

## Hand Scrunches

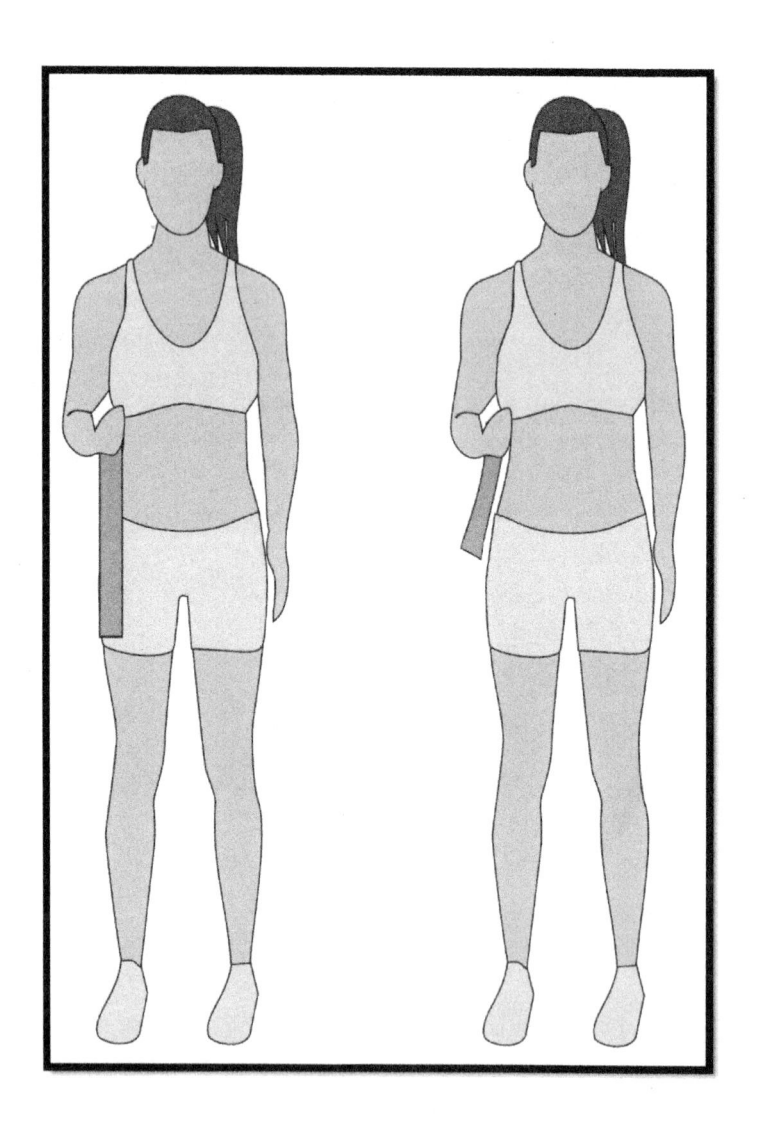

# Exercises with Resistance Loop Bands (2nd Edition)

*Effect:* This exercise works on strengthening of the hand muscles.

*Difficulty Level:* Beginner

*Start Position:* Hold the loop band in your hand.

*Steps:*

1. Scrunch the band in your hand and release.
2. Repeat it 10 times.

## Bear Crawls

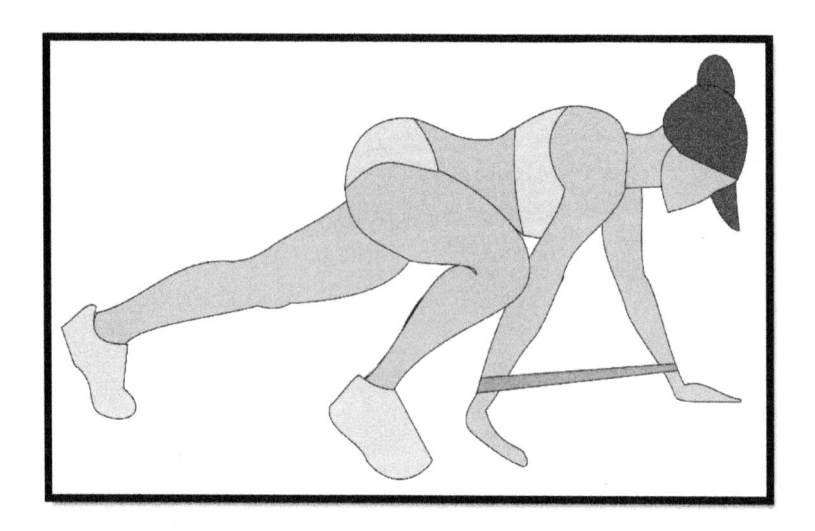

# Exercises with Resistance Loop Bands (2nd Edition)

*Effect:* This is a full body mobility exercise which works on strengthening of your arm muscles.

*Difficulty Level:* Advanced

*Start Position:* Put the resistance band around your wrists and come in all fours position with your hands under the shoulder and knees under the hips.

*Steps:*

1. Start crawling, moving your left hand and right leg forward and vice-versa, maintaining shoulders and hips in one horizontal plane.
2. Always maintain tension in the loop band.
3. You can move forwards, sidewards and backwards to have variation in the exercise.

*Fine Tips:*

1. Keep shoulders and hips in one horizontal plane throughout the movement.
2. Always maintain a slight tension in the band; a slack band would tend to slide down interfering in your exercise.

## Lateral Arm Raise (Rotator Cuff)

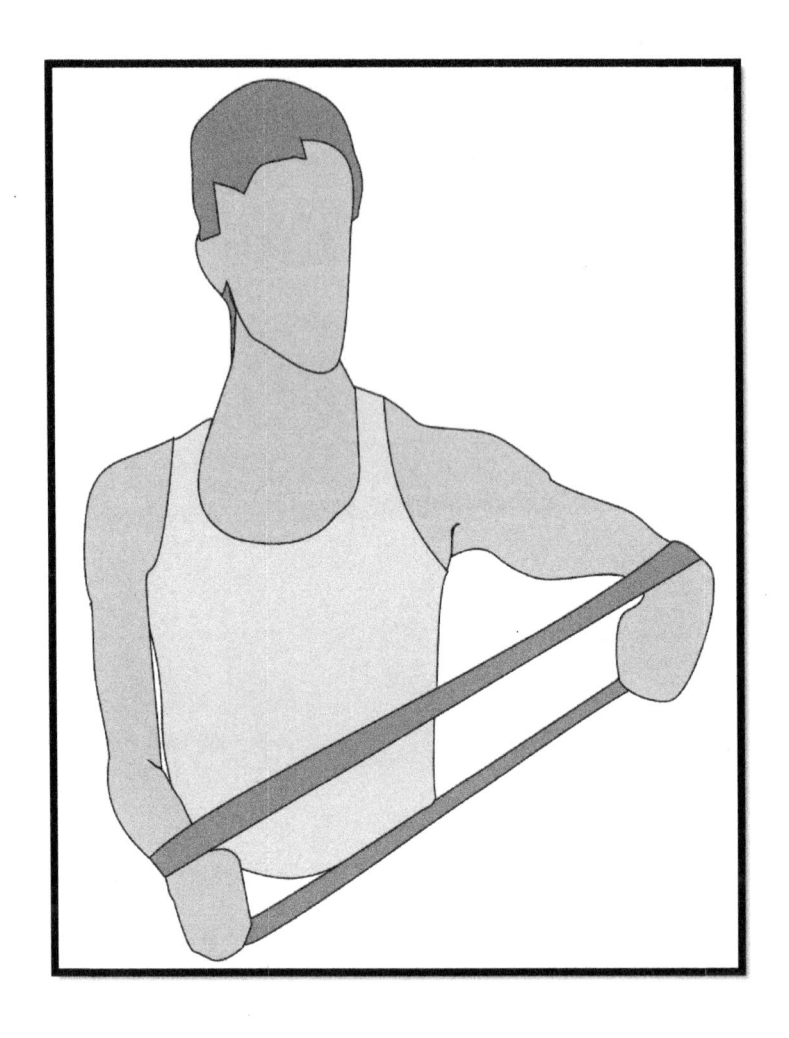

# Exercises with Resistance Loop Bands (2nd Edition)

*Effect:* This exercise works on strengthening of shoulder and arm abductor and internal rotator muscles.

*Difficulty Level:* Advanced

*Start Position:* Stand tall with back straight, abdomen tucked in and feet hip width distance apart. Bend the arms at 90 degrees to the elbows and tuck them by the side of your trunk.

*Steps:*

1. Place the resistance band around your wrists. Putting outward pressure on both the ends of the band, raise your left arm laterally upwards, maintaining the 90 degree bend at elbow.
2. Hold the left arm in fully stretched position for 5 counts.
3. Release the stretch slowly, getting left arm back to the starting position.
4. Repeat required number of times.
5. Repeat on the right side.

*Fine Tips:*

1. Keep your shoulders down throughout the movement.

## Seated Concentration Curl

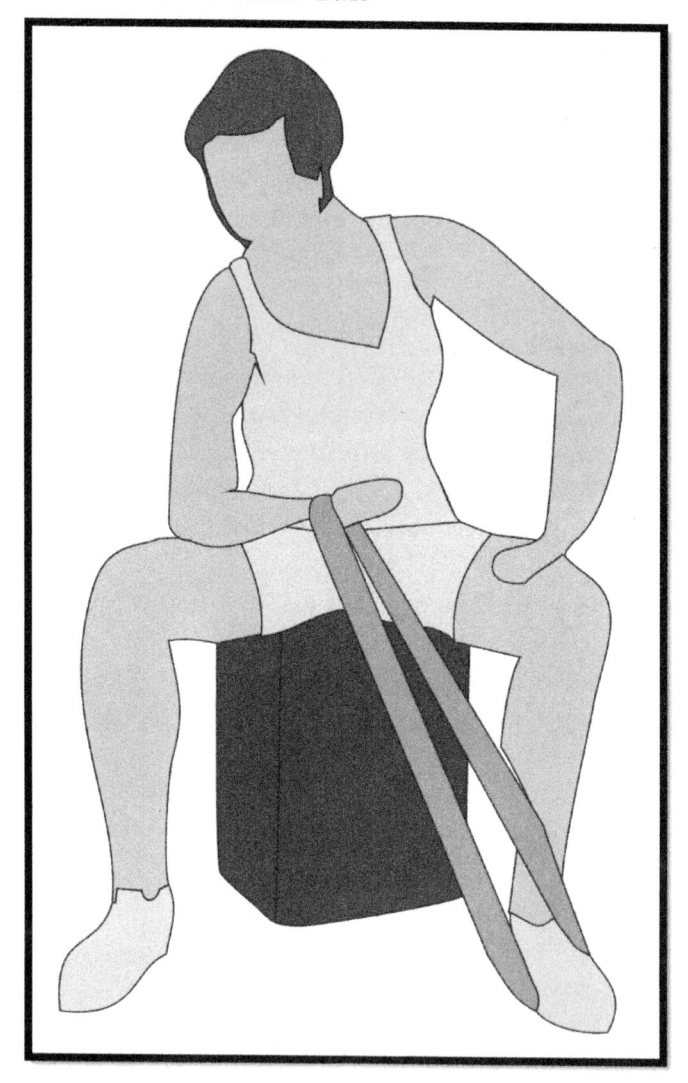

# Exercises with Resistance Loop Bands (2nd Edition)

*Effect:* This exercise works on strengthening of biceps, brachialis and brachioradialis muscles.

*Difficulty Level:* Beginner

*Start Position:* Sit on a bench, placing resistance loop around left foot and grasp the band with an up grip in your right hand.

*Steps:*

1. Sit with your abdomen tucked in and bend your elbow to bring the band towards your chest.
2. Squeeze the biceps at the fully contracted position. Hold for 5 counts.
3. Release the stretch and return to the start position slowly.
4. Do the required number of repetitions.
5. Repeat on the other side.

*Fine Tips:*

1. There should be no movement at the upper torso throughout the exercise.

Dr. Monika Chopra's Fitness Sutra

## Wrist Curl

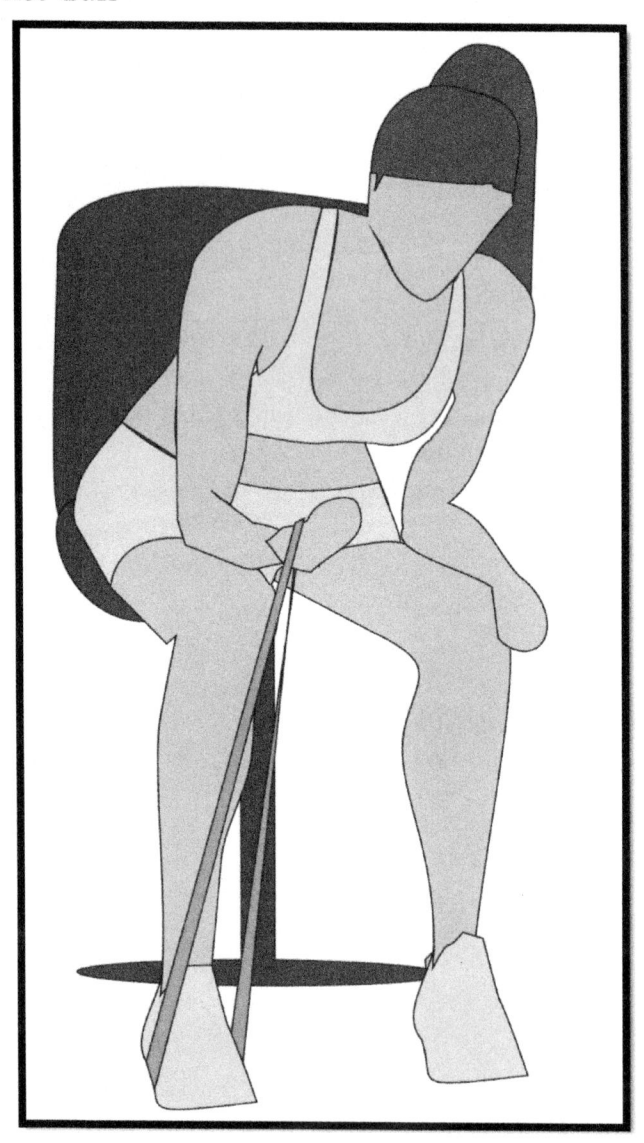

*Effect:* This exercise works on strengthening of front forearm muscles.

*Difficulty Level:* Beginner

*Start Position:* Sit on a chair. Put the resistance band around your right foot and hold the band in your right hand in up grip with your forearms resting on respective thighs.

*Steps:*

1. Bend your wrist, pulling the band up.
2. Feel the muscles of your front right forearm contracting. Hold the stretched position for 5 counts.
3. Release the stretch and return the wrist to the start position.
4. Do required number of repetitions.
5. Repeat with other wrist.

*Fine Tips:*

1. Keep your forearm stable and supported throughout the movement.
2. The movement should be slow and controlled.

*"We make our destiny and we call it fate"*

— *Benjamin Disraeli*

# CHAPTER 5

Lower Body Exercises

## Bridge Thrust

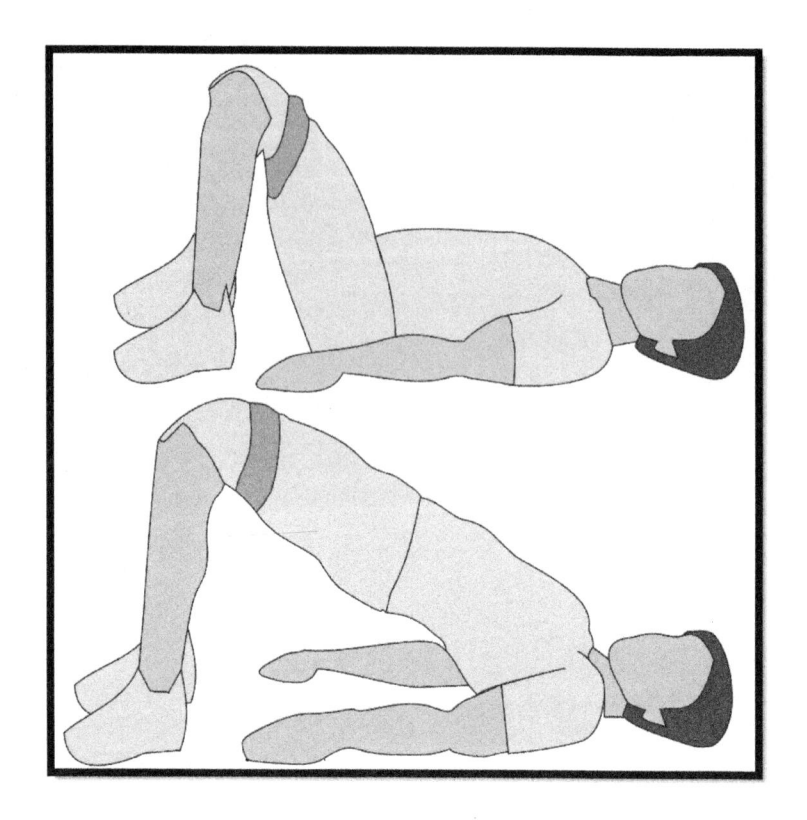

# Exercises with Resistance Loop Bands (2nd Edition)

*Effect:* This exercise helps in strengthening of the gluteal muscles.

*Difficulty Level:* Advanced

*Start Position:* Lie down straight on your back with legs bent at knee, feet flat on the floor, shoulder width apart and hands by the side of your body. Place the resistance band around your thighs, just above the knees.

*Steps:*

1. Exhale and imprint your back on the floor.
2. Inhale and raise your hips up till your back, hips and thighs come in one line.
3. Hold this position for 5 seconds (keep breathing as you hold the position).
4. Slowly release the position and get your hips down back to the start position as you exhale.
5. Repeat required number of times.

*Fine Tips:*

1. Keep tension in the loop band throughout the exercise.
2. Keep breathing throughout the exercise.

## One Leg Hip Thrust

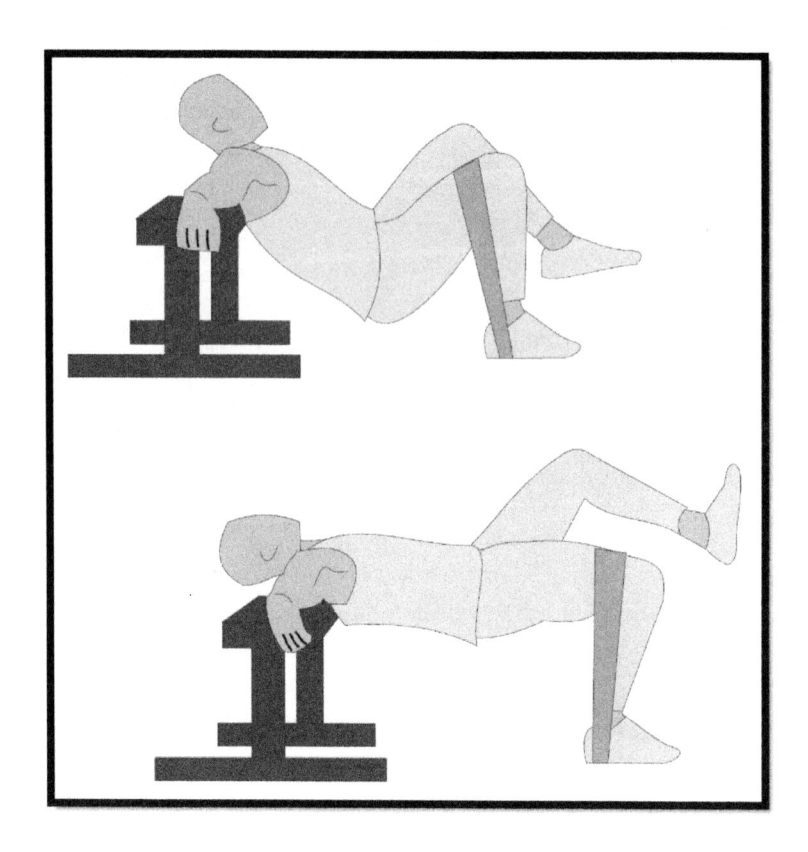

*Effect:* This exercise helps to strengthen the gluteal and hip extensor muscles.

*Difficulty Level:* Advanced

*Start Position:* Wrap the resistance loop band around the bottom of your right foot and around the right thigh. Sit on the ground with feet flat on the floor, arms externally rotated and raised to shoulder level, arms and back rested against the bench. The left leg is partially flexed and raised in the air.

*Steps:*

1. Push down through the right heel and slowly raise your hips up, till your right knee, hip and shoulder come in one line, parallel to the floor.
2. Hold this position for 5 seconds.
3. Slowly lower down the hips, returning to the start position.
4. Repeat required number of times.
5. Repeat on the other side.

*Fine Tips:*

1. Let your torso and head follow the hip raise and feel the glutes contract as you do the movement.
2. The movement should be slow and controlled keeping the hips squared.

## Side Step Squats

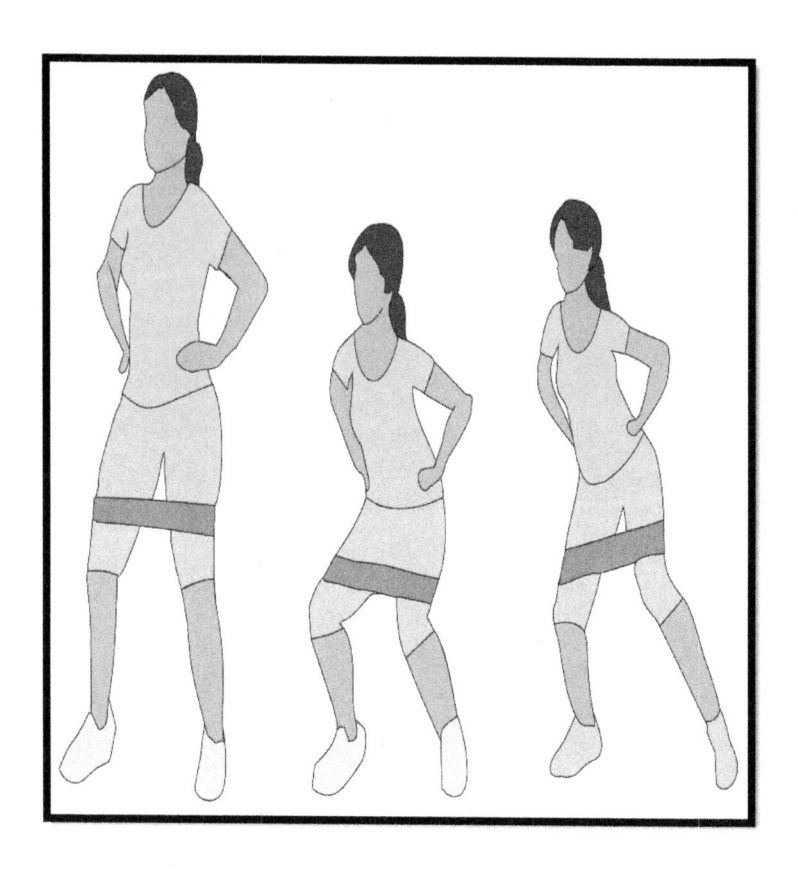

*Effect:* This exercise works on strengthening of leg abductors and quadriceps muscles.

*Difficulty Level:* Advanced

*Start Position:* Loop the resistance band around your lower thigh just above the knees. Stand with feet shoulder width apart.

*Steps:*

1. Move the left leg horizontally sidewards as if taking a side step. Go in squat position and hold there for 5 counts.
2. Release the stretch and come back to start position.
3. Repeat it on the right side.

*Fine Tips:*

1. Do not squat above 90 degrees as you do the movement.

## Lying Hip Abduction

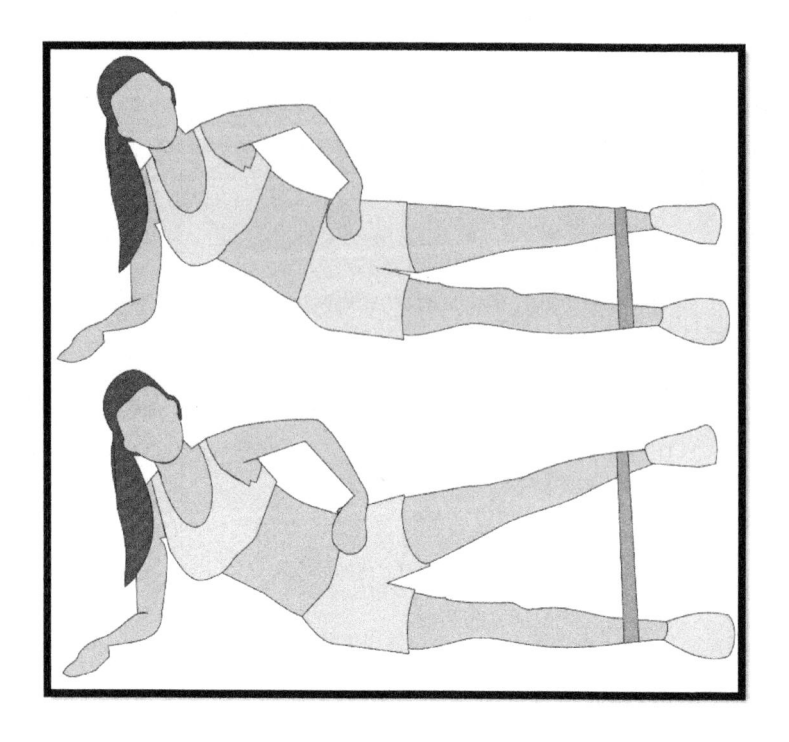

*Effect:* This exercise helps in strengthening of leg abductor muscles.

*Difficulty Level:* Advanced

*Start Position:* Put the resistance loop around your ankles. Lie on your right side, supporting your torso on the arm, bent at 90 degrees at elbow. Your upper leg is above your lower leg, hip width apart.

*Steps:*

1. Raise your left leg up, pulling the resistance band. Hold the left leg at maximum stretch position for 5 counts (without changing the form).
2. Slowly lower the left leg to start position.
3. Do required number of repetitions.
4. Repeat on the other side.

*Fine Tips:*

1. Keep your knee slightly flexed (do not hyperextend the knee) as you do the movement.
2. Maintain your body in straight line (do not bend forwards or backwards with the movement).

## Lying Leg Raise

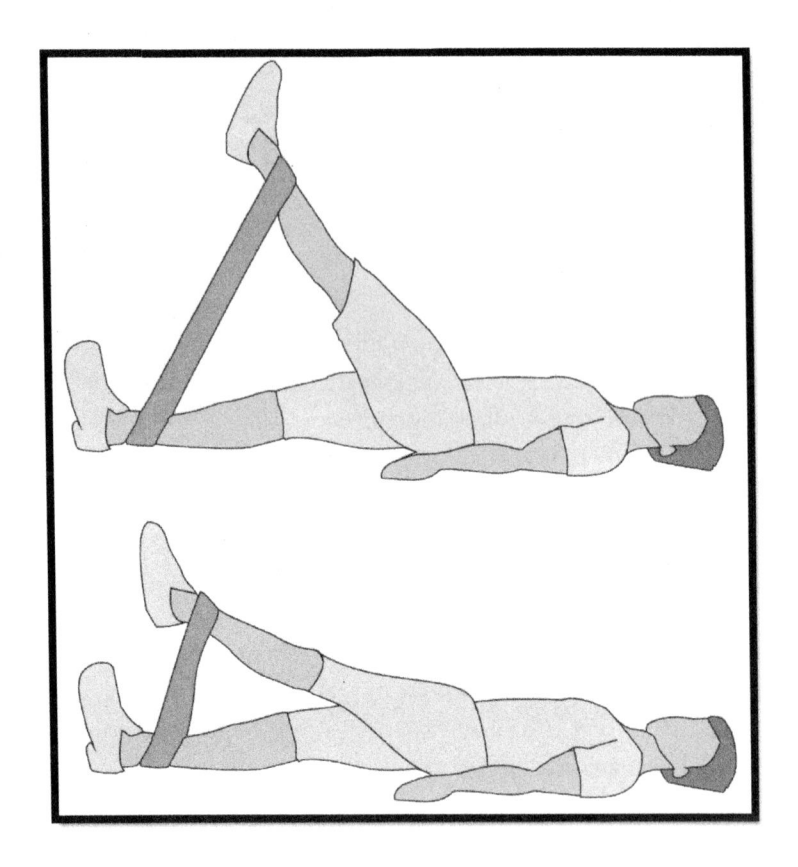

# Exercises with Resistance Loop Bands (2nd Edition)

*Effect:* This exercise works on strengthening of hip flexor muscles.

*Difficulty Level:* Beginner

*Start Position:* Put the resistance loop around your ankle. Lie down on your back with left leg over the right and arms by the side of your body.

*Steps:*

1. Tuck your abdominals in as you exhale.
2. Inhale and lift your left leg up, to the maximum band stretch position. Hold the leg up for 5 counts. Keep breathing.
3. Exhale and slowly get the leg down to start position.
4. Do required number of repetitions.
5. Repeat with right leg.

*Fine Tips:*

1. Maintain the imprinting of your back as you perform the movement.
2. Do not hyperextend your leg anytime during the movement.

## Standing Hip Abduction

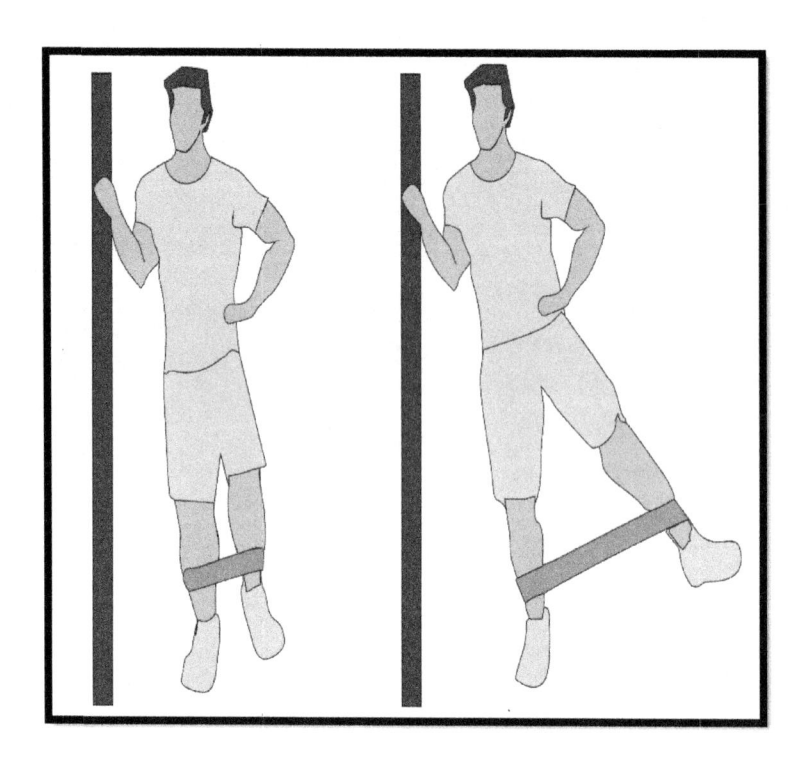

# Exercises with Resistance Loop Bands (2nd Edition)

*Effect:* This exercise works on strengthening of the hip abductor muscles

*Difficulty Level:* Beginner

*Start Position:* Put the resistance loop around your ankle. Stand tall with the right side of your body next to the wall and feet hip width distance apart.

*Steps:*

1. Squeeze your right glutes and stand on the right foot. Start raising your left leg sideways upwards pulling the resistance loop apart. Feel your left abductors contracting.
2. Hold your leg up in maximum stretch position for 5 counts.
3. Slowly bring the leg back to start position as you release the stretch.
4. Perform the required number of repetitions and then repeat with the other leg.

*Fine Tips:*

1. Do not tilt on the supporting leg side as you raise the other leg.
2. Keep the supporting leg glutes contracted throughout the movement
3. Keep both the knees slightly flexed as you do the movement.

## Band Squats

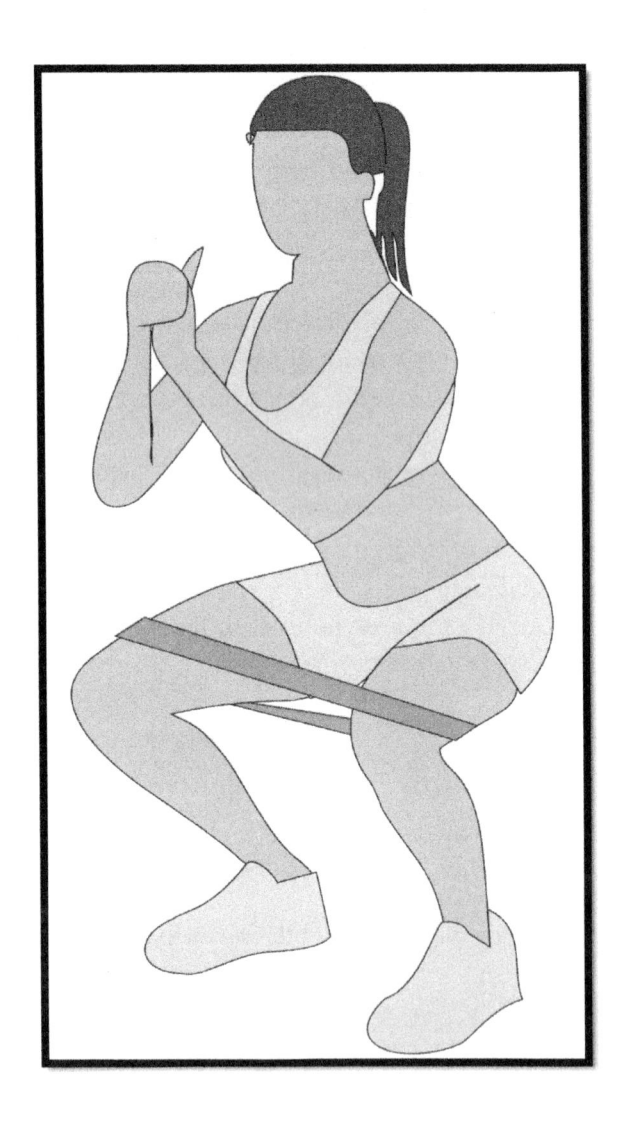

*Effect:* This exercise works on strengthening of the quadriceps and hip abductor muscles.

*Difficulty Level:* Advanced

*Start Position:* Stand with the resistance loop band around your thighs, just above the knees. Move your feet shoulder width apart, with chest and head up.

*Steps:*

1. Sit your hips back, bending at the knee. Push your knees out and against the resistance loop as you squat, getting your thighs parallel to the floor.
2. Once your thighs are parallel to the floor, hold the position for 5 counts.
3. Push through your heels and come up to the starting position.
4. Do required number of repetitions.

*Fine Tips:*

1. Maintain your upper body form as you do the movement.
2. Do not squat above 90 degrees.

## Leg Extension

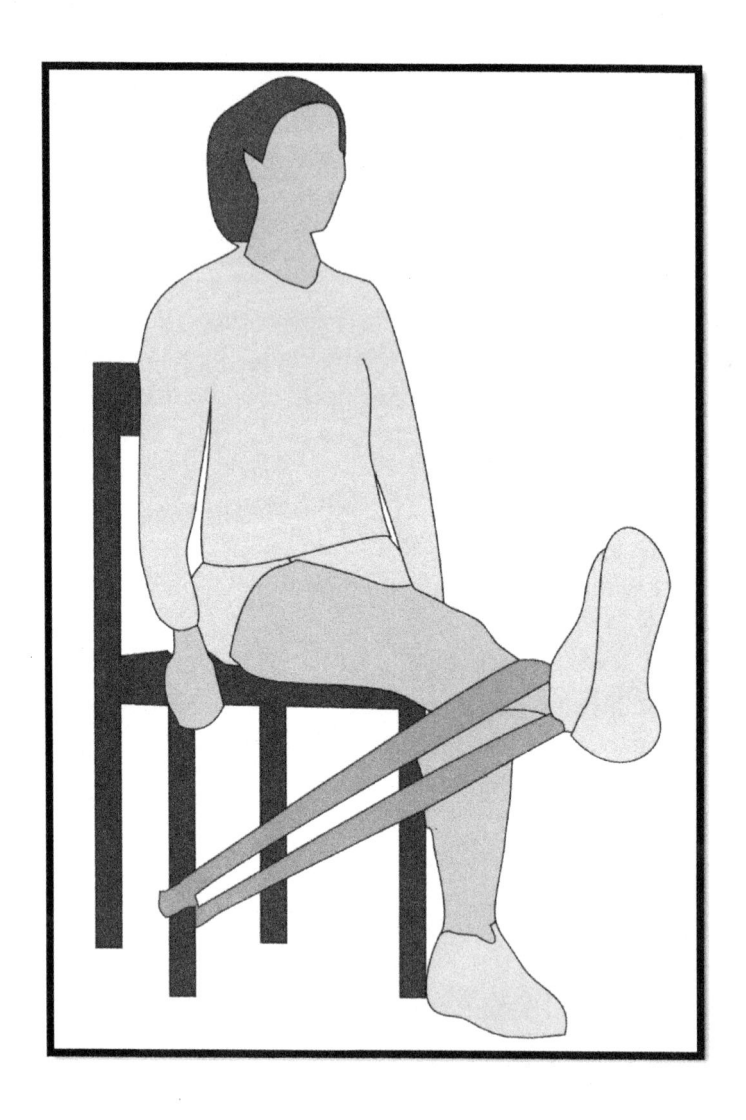

# Exercises with Resistance Loop Bands (2nd Edition)

*Effect:* This exercise works on strengthening of the quadriceps muscles.

*Difficulty Level:* Beginner

*Start Position:* Sit tall on the chair, with abdomen tucked in, feet hip width distance apart and flat on the ground. Place one end of the band in leg of the chair and other end over your right ankle.

*Steps:*

1. Hold the base of the chair with your hands as you raise the right leg against the resistance of the band. Raise it till it comes in line with thigh. Contract your front thigh muscle as you raise the leg.
2. Hold the leg in this position for 5 counts.
3. Slowly lower the leg down to the start position as you release the stretch.
4. Perform the required number of repetitions.
5. Repeat on the other side.

*Fine Tips:*

1. Do not take your upper body back as you raise the leg.
2. Do not hyper extend the knee of the raised leg.
3. Your thighs should rest on the chair throughout the movement.

## Clam Shell

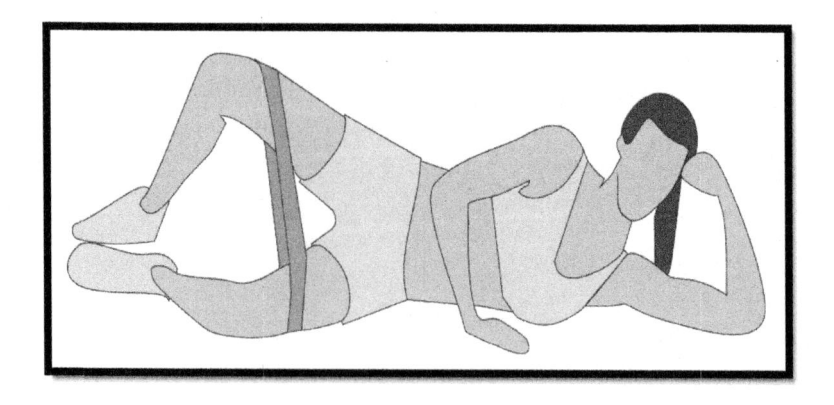

*Effect:* This exercise helps in strengthening of hip abductors and external rotator muscles.

*Difficulty Level:* Advanced

*Start Position:* Slide the resistance loop above the knees. Lie in the side lying position, with your right knee above the left, your right feet above the left, hips slightly bent, knees bent at 90 degrees and ankles touching each other. Your upper body should be supported by right hand, placed flat in front of the upper body.

*Steps:*

1. Keeping your feet together raise your right knee up (taking right leg in external rotation), right thigh pushing against the resistance loop band.
2. Pause at the top for a second and slowly move the right knee down to the starting position.
3. After required number of repetitions, repeat on the left side.

*Fine Tips:*

1. Keep your body (especially pelvis and left leg) stable and in start form as you rotate the leg.

# Thigh Thrust

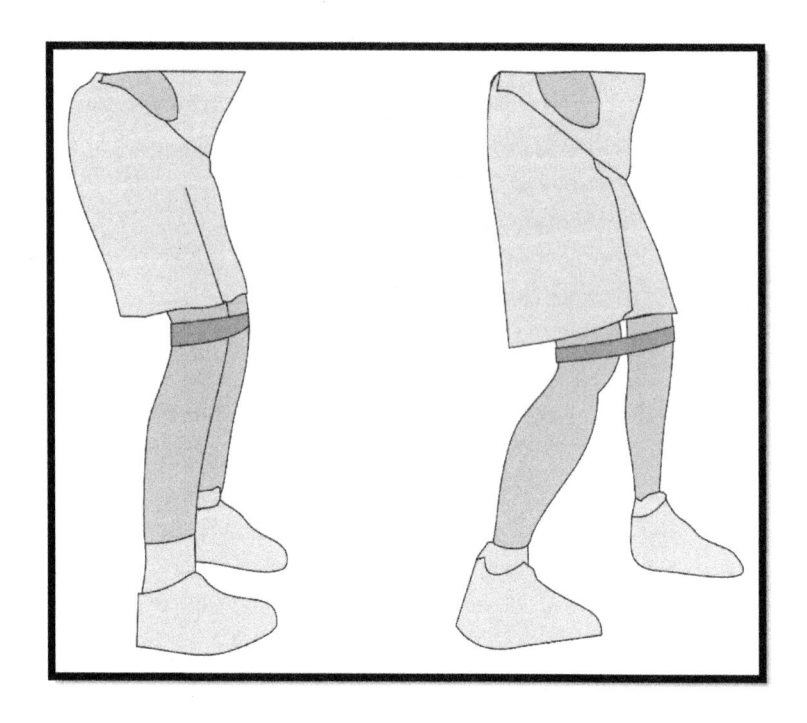

## Exercises with Resistance Loop Bands (2nd E

*Effect:* This exercise helps in strengthe
leg muscles.

*Difficulty Level:* Beginner

*Start Position:* Loop the resistance band above your knees and stand with feet hip width distance apart. The band should be stretched.

*Steps:*

1. Resist the pull of the band as you take five steps forward.
2. Continue to resist the pull of the band as you take five steps back.
3. You can repeat this exercise walking sideways.

*Fine Tips:*

1. Keep your knees slightly flexed (bent) as you perform the movement.

## Lateral Walk

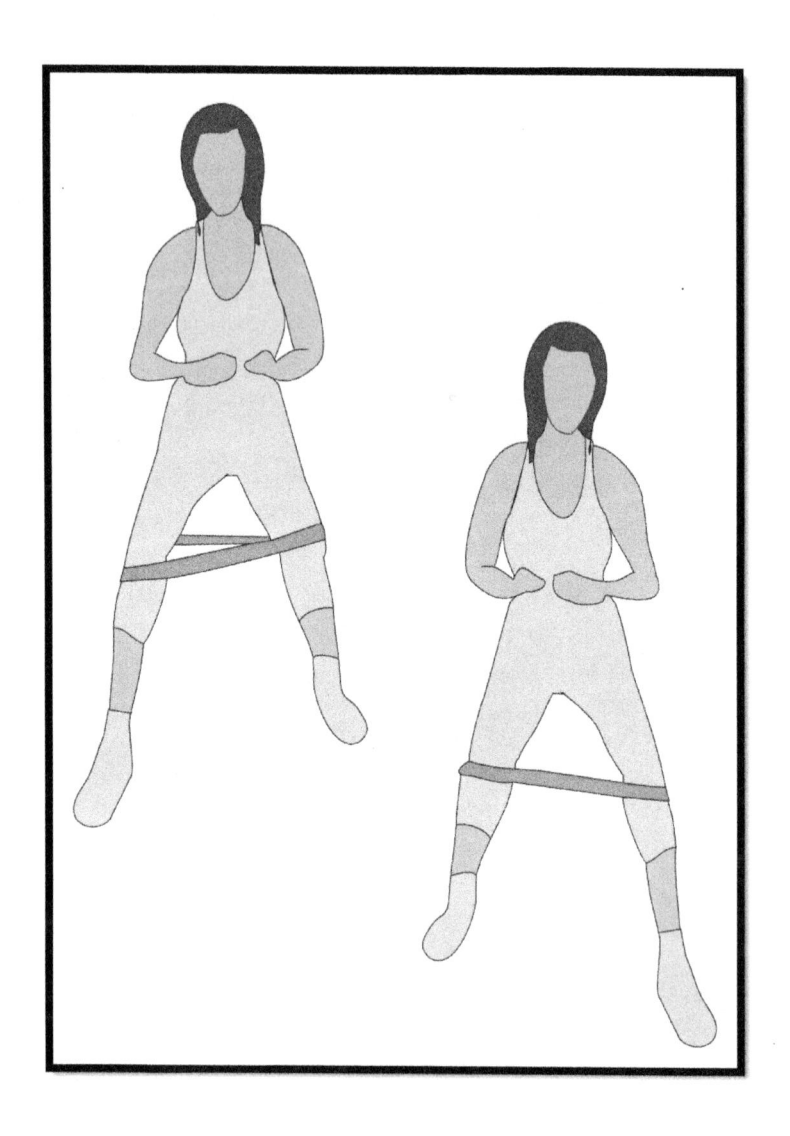

# Exercises with Resistance Loop Bands (2nd Edition)

*Effect:* This exercise helps in strengthening of leg muscles.

*Difficulty Level:* Beginner

*Start Position:* Stand with feet shoulder width apart and resistance loop band around the lower thigh, just above the knees. Create tension in the band. Bend at your knees, keeping the back tall.

*Steps:*

1. Take an exaggerated step to the right to maximally stretch out the loop band. Continue in that direction for 5 steps.
2. Take five exaggerated steps to the left to return to the start position. Repeat on the other side.

*Fine Tips:*

1. Keep your back tall and knees slightly flexed as you do the movement.

## Standing Hip Flexion

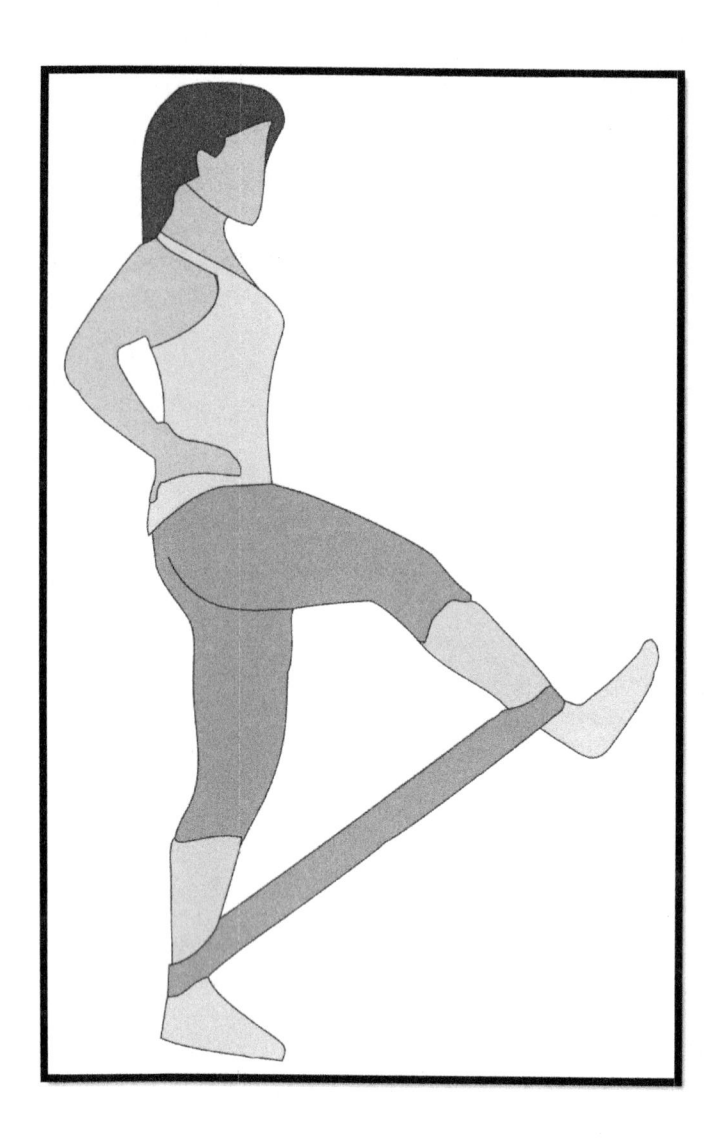

*Effect:* This exercise helps in strengthening of the hip flexor muscles.

*Difficulty Level:* Advanced

*Start Position:* Stand tall with feet hip width distance apart and the resistance loop band around the ankles.

*Steps:*

1. Shifting your weight to the left leg, raise your right leg forward, pulling the band.
2. Hold the stretched position for 5 counts and return to the start position.
3. Perform required number of repetitions.
4. Repeat on the other side.

*Fine Tips:*

1. Keep your torso tall throughout the movement.
2. Never lock (hyperextend) the knees.

## Single Leg Loop Bridge

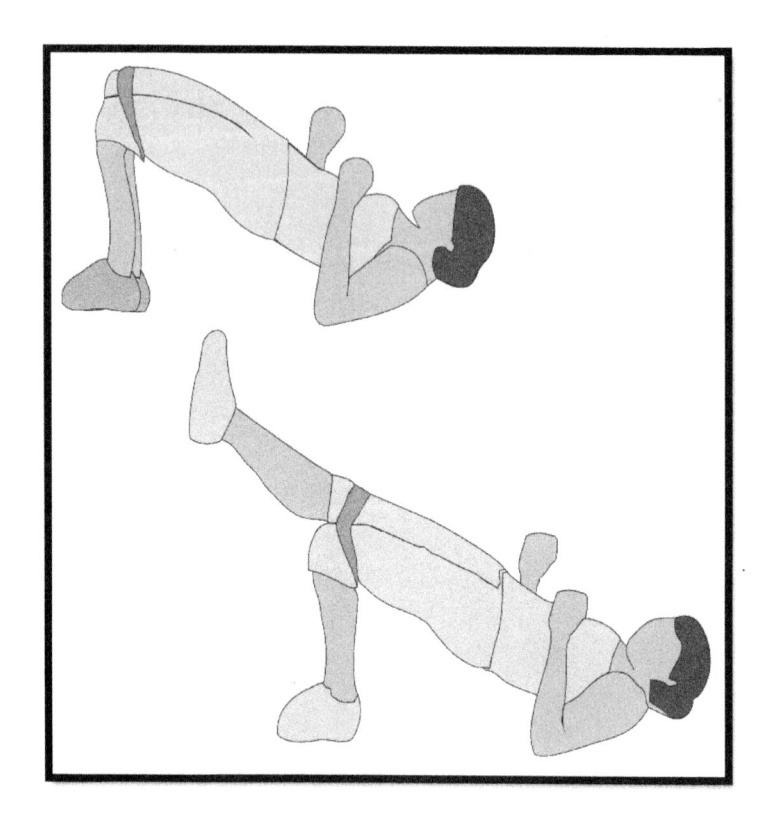

# Exercises with Resistance Loop Bands (2nd Edition)

*Effect:* This exercise helps in strengthening of glutes and quadriceps muscles.

*Difficulty Level:* Advanced

*Start Position:* Loop the resistance band around your lower thigh, just above the knees. Lie down in bridge position (feet flat on the floor, arms by your sides, abdomen braced and hips lifted up with glutes contracted).

*Steps:*

1. Raise your right leg up, keeping thigh in line with thigh and pull your toes towards you. Hold this position for 5 counts.
2. Slowly lower down the leg to start position.
3. Perform required number of times.
4. Repeat on the other side.

*Fine Tips:*

1. Keep the knees together and maintain the bridge position throughout the exercise.
2. Do not hyperextend the knee of the straight leg.

# Dr. Monika Chopra's Fitness Sutra

## Backwards Leg Swing

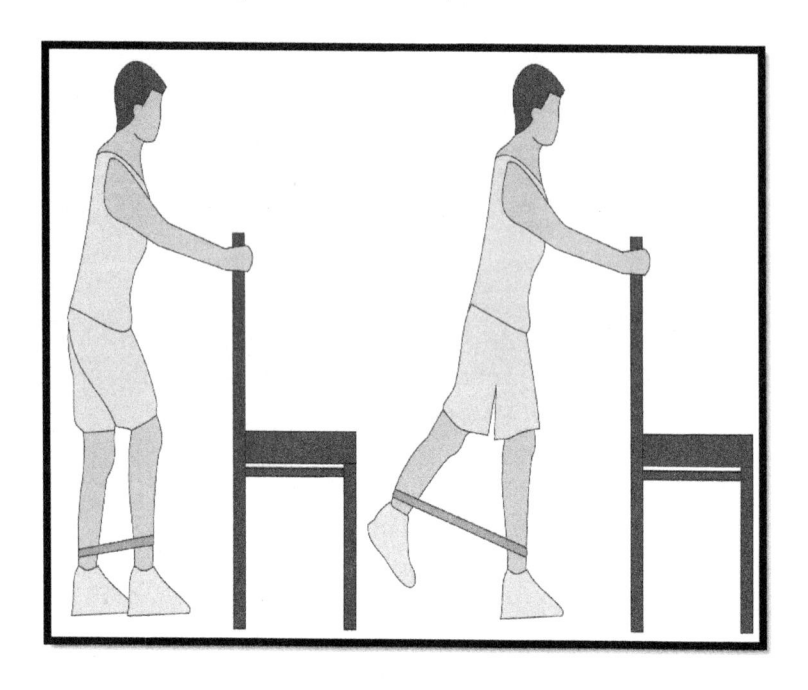

# Exercises with Resistance Loop Bands (2nd E

*Effect:* This exercise helps in strength extensor muscles.

*Difficulty Level:* Beginner

*Start Position:* Stand tall with feet hip width distance apart, facing a chair and put one or both hand on the chair to balance. Put the resistance loop band around your ankles. You may put one end of the loop around right ankle and other end under the left heel to stabilize it.

*Steps:*

1. Shift your weight to left leg keeping your abdominals engaged and glutes contracted. Take the right leg behind stretching the band to maximum.
2. Hold for 5 counts.
3. Slowly get the right leg back to the start position.
4. Perform required number of repetitions.
5. Repeat on the other side.

*Fine Tips:*

1. Keep your torso tall throughout the exercise.

## Standing Hip Adduction

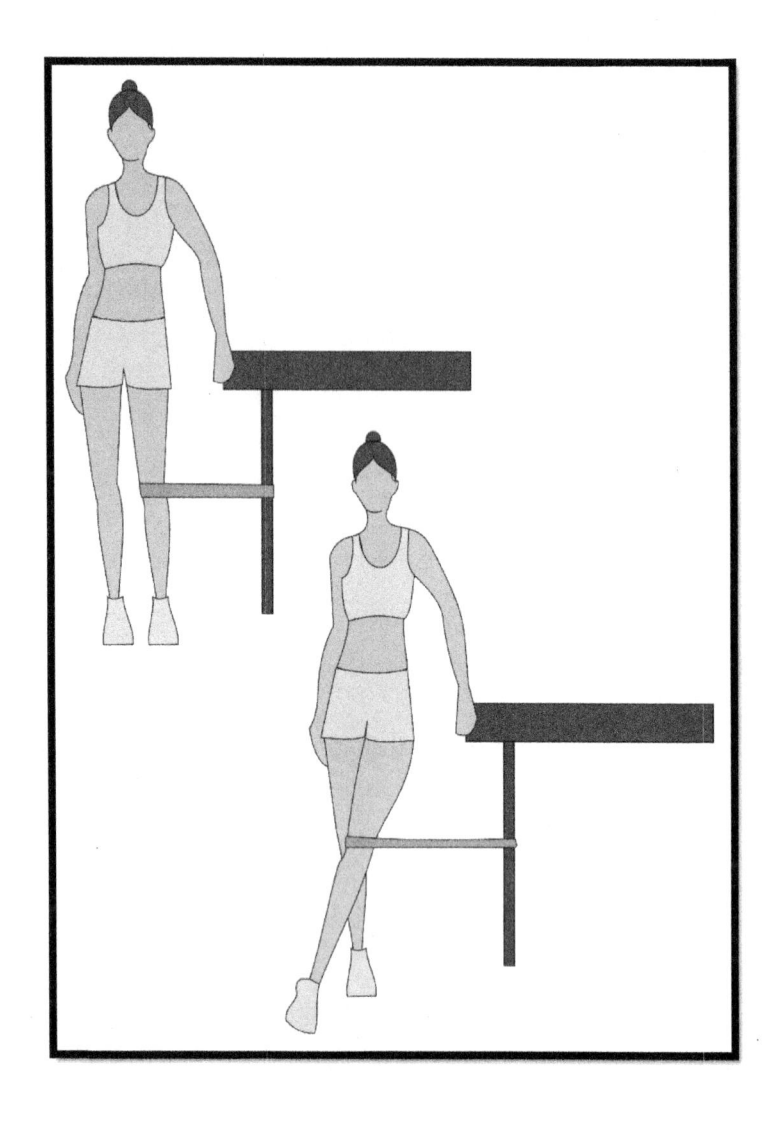

# Exercises with Resistance Loop Bands (2nd Edition)

*Effect:* This exercise helps to strengthen the ...r adductor muscles.

*Difficulty Level:* Beginner

*Start Position:* Stand tall by the side of a table or pole (which is on the left side of your body). The distance between leg and table or pole should be around 1 feet. Loop the band around the left thigh and the leg of the table.

*Steps:*

1. Lift your left leg out to the right side till it comes off the ground.
2. Hold the leg with maximum band stretch position for 5 second and then slowly get it back to the start position.
3. Perform the required number of repetitions.
4. Repeat on the other side.

*Fine Tips:*

1. You can hold onto the furniture or the wall to maintain balance while taking the leg side wards, away from the table/pole.
2. Keep your torso tall throughout the movement.
3. Keep the moving leg straight with toes pointing forward as you do the movement.

## Standing Hip Extension

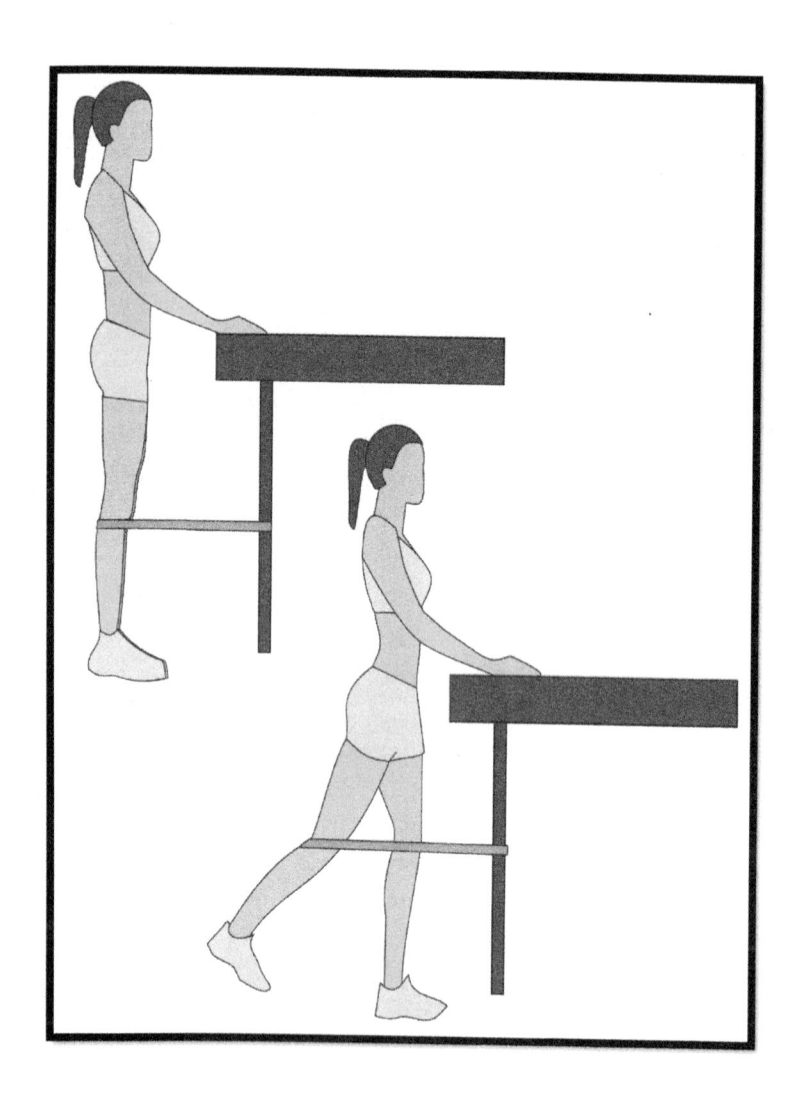

# Exercises with Resistance Loop Bands (2nd Edit

*Effect:* This exercise helps in strengthening of hip extensor muscles.

*Difficulty Level:* Beginner

*Start Position:* Loop the band around your right leg and the leg of a table or a pole. Stand tall facing the table, with your abdomen tucked in and feet hip width distance apart.

*Steps:*
1. Keeping your leg straight and toes pointing forwards, push your leg backwards till it comes slightly above the ground.
2. Hold the leg with band in maximum stretch for 5 counts and return to the start position.
3. Perform the required number of repetitions.
4. Repeat on the other side.

*Fine Tips:*
1. You can hold onto the furniture or wall to maintain the balance, as you raise your leg.

## Seated Leg Extension

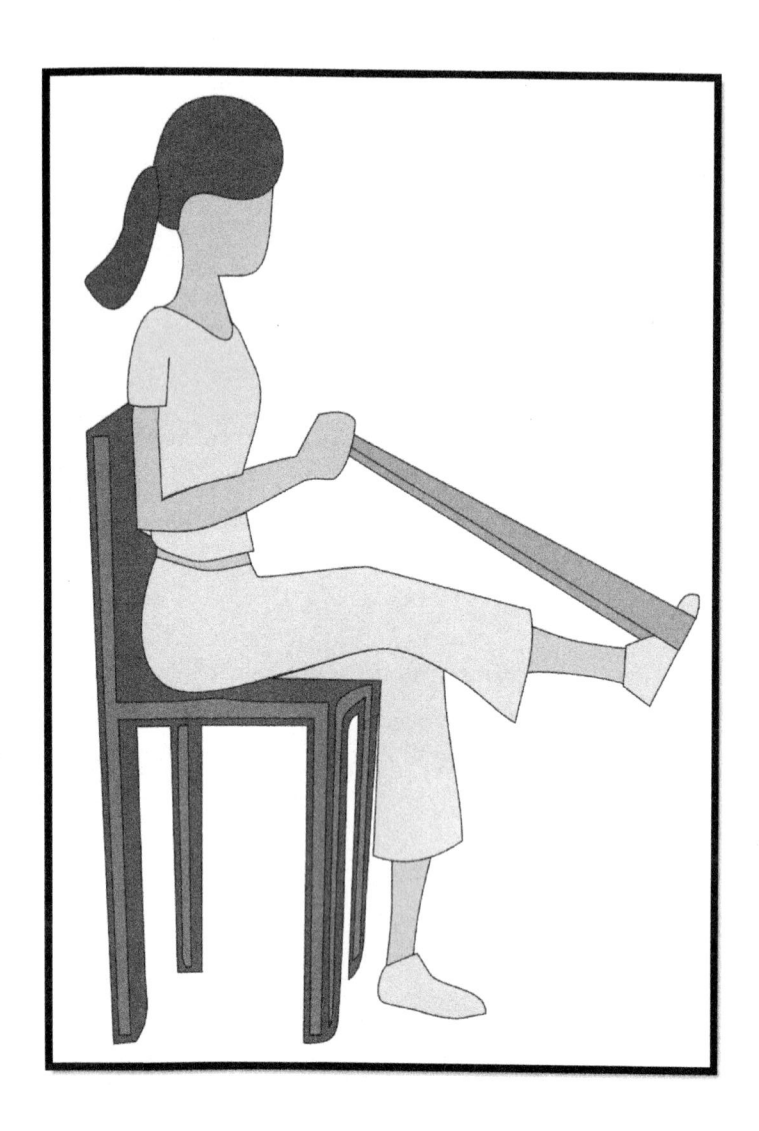

# Exercises with Resistance Loop Bands (2nd Edition)

*Effect:* This exercise helps in strengthening of knee extensor muscles .

*Difficulty Level:* Advanced

*Start Position:* Sit on the chair with back tall and supported. Put the loop band around your right foot.

*Steps:*

1. Hold the band in the right hand and extend your leg against the resistance of loop band.
2. Hold for 5 counts and then release, getting it back to the start position.
3. Perform required number of repetitions on each leg.

*Fine Tips:*

1. Keep the knee of the extended leg slightly flexed (avoid knee hyperextension) in the up position.

Dr. Monika Chopra's Fitness Sutra

## Seated Hip Abduction

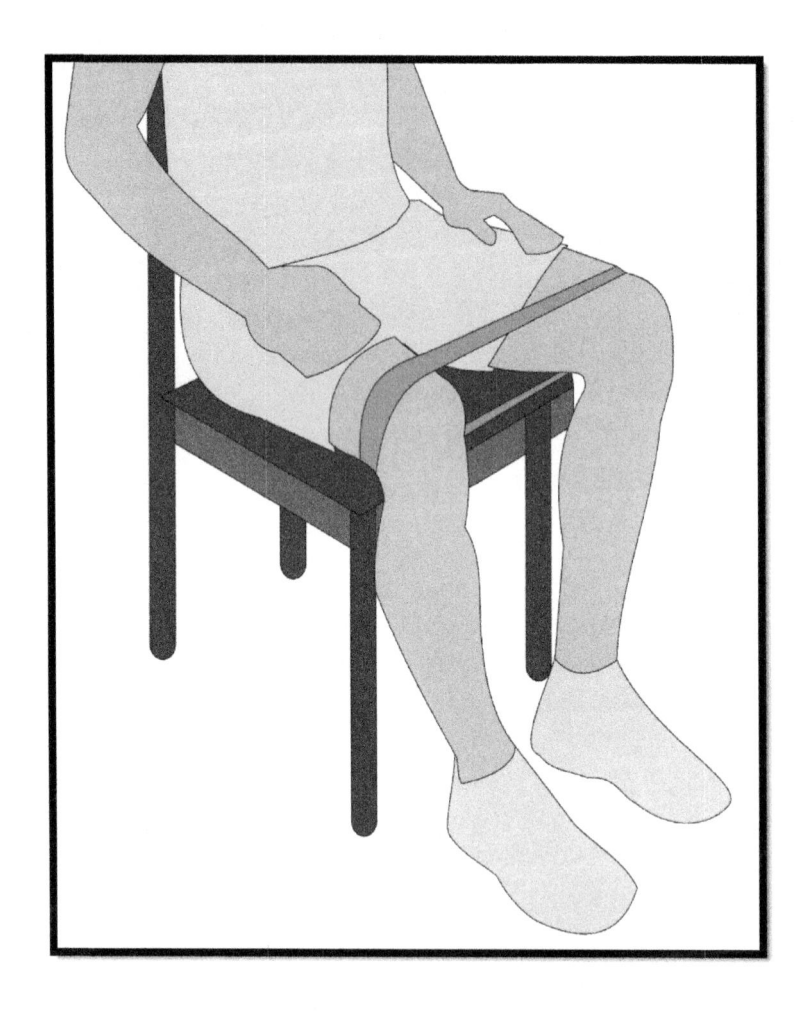

# Exercises with Resistance Loop Bands (2nd Edition)

*Effect:* This exercise helps in strengthening of hip abductor muscles.

*Difficulty Level:* Beginner

*Start Position:* Loop the resistance band around your thigh and sit tall on the chair with feet grounded.

*Steps:*

1. Push your legs out to the sides, so that the band stretches.
2. Hold for 5 counts.
3. Return to the start position.
4. Perform required number of repetitions.

## Ankle Internal Rotation

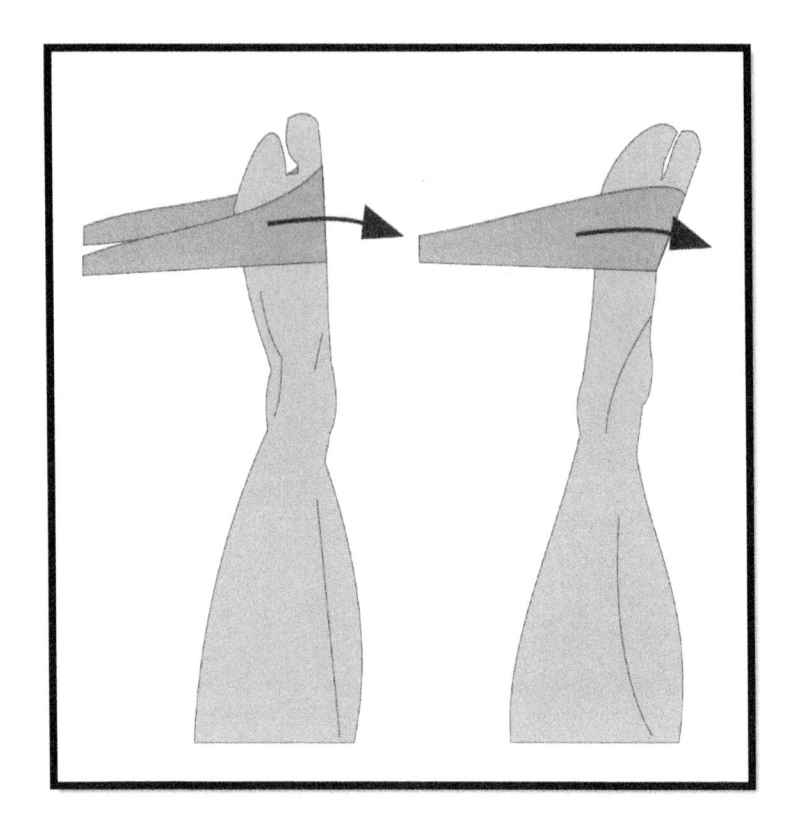

# Exercises with Resistance Loop Bands (2nd Edition)

*Effect:* This exercise helps in strengthening of the leg internal rotator muscles.

*Difficulty Level:* Beginner

*Start Position:* Wrap the resistance loop band around your forefoot and sit on the floor in a long sitting position with your legs extended in front. Tie the loop band on the other side to a fixed support.

*Steps:*

1. Keeping the leg at the same place rotate your leg inwards, moving the foot away from the fixed support with the band resisting the movement.
2. Hold the foot in maximum band stretch position for 5 counts
3. Slowly rotate the foot back to the start position.
4. Repeat it required number of times.
5. Repeat on the other side.

*Fine Tips:*

1. Rotate the whole leg as you do the movement.

## Supinated Clamshell

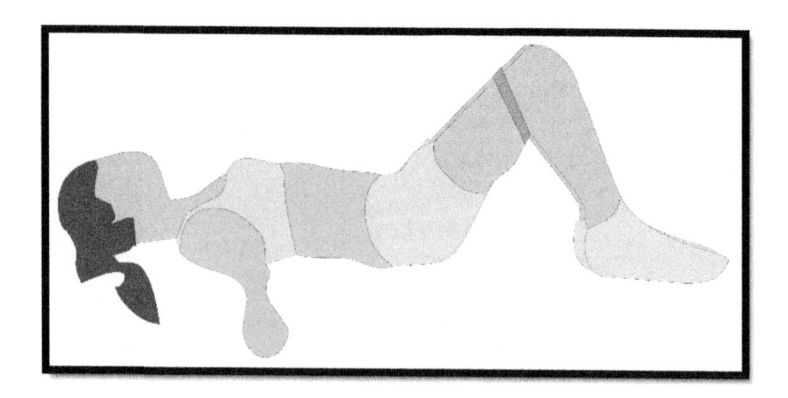

*Effect:* This exercise helps to strengthen the hip abductors and external rotator muscles.

*Difficulty Level:* Beginner

*Start Position:* Put the resistance loop around your thighs just above the knees. Lie down on your back with hips and knees flexed (knees flexed at 90 degrees), legs shoulder width distance apart and abdomen tucked in.

*Steps:*

1. Pull the knees apart while contracting your glutes.
2. Hold for 5 seconds.
3. Slowly get the knees back to the start position.
4. Perform the required number of repetitions.

# CHAPTER 6

Chest & Back Exercises

## Lateral Push Up

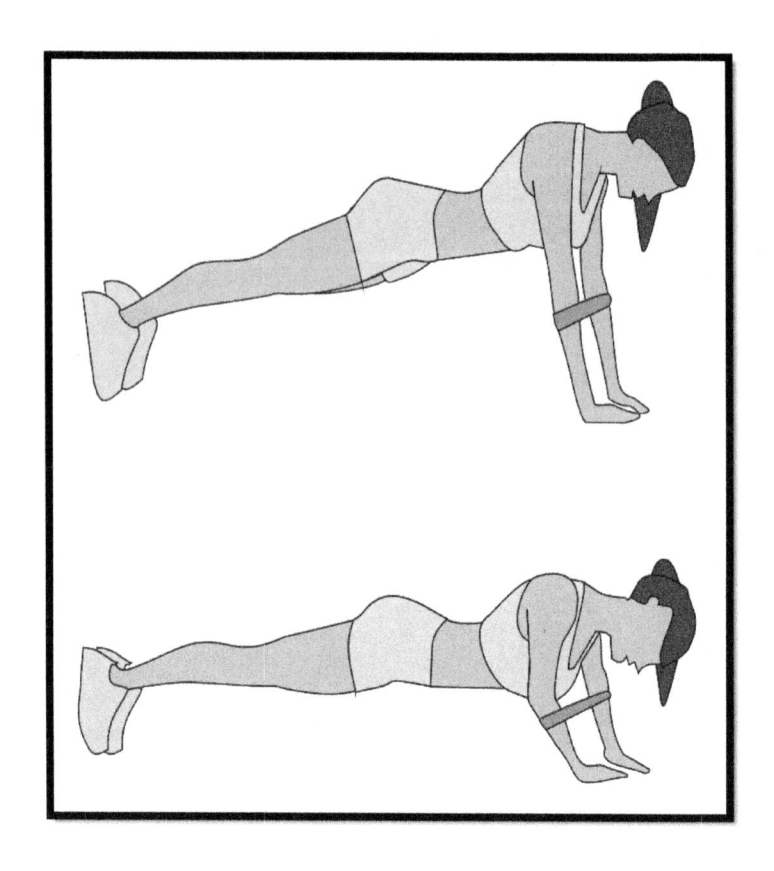

*Effect:* This exercise helps in strengthening of shoulder and arm muscles.

*Difficulty Level:* Advanced

*Start Position:* Come in plank position with arms extended and hands shoulder width apart. Put the resistance loop band around the arms.

*Steps:*

1. Go down on the hands, bending the arms at elbows, with the lateral side of arms pushing against the band.
2. Hold down position for 5 counts and come back to the start position.
3. Perform required number of repetitions.

*Fine Tips:*

1. Maintain the straight body form with movement occurring only at the arms as you take the body up and down on the arms.

# Dr. Monika Chopra's Fitness Sutra

## Lateral Pull Down

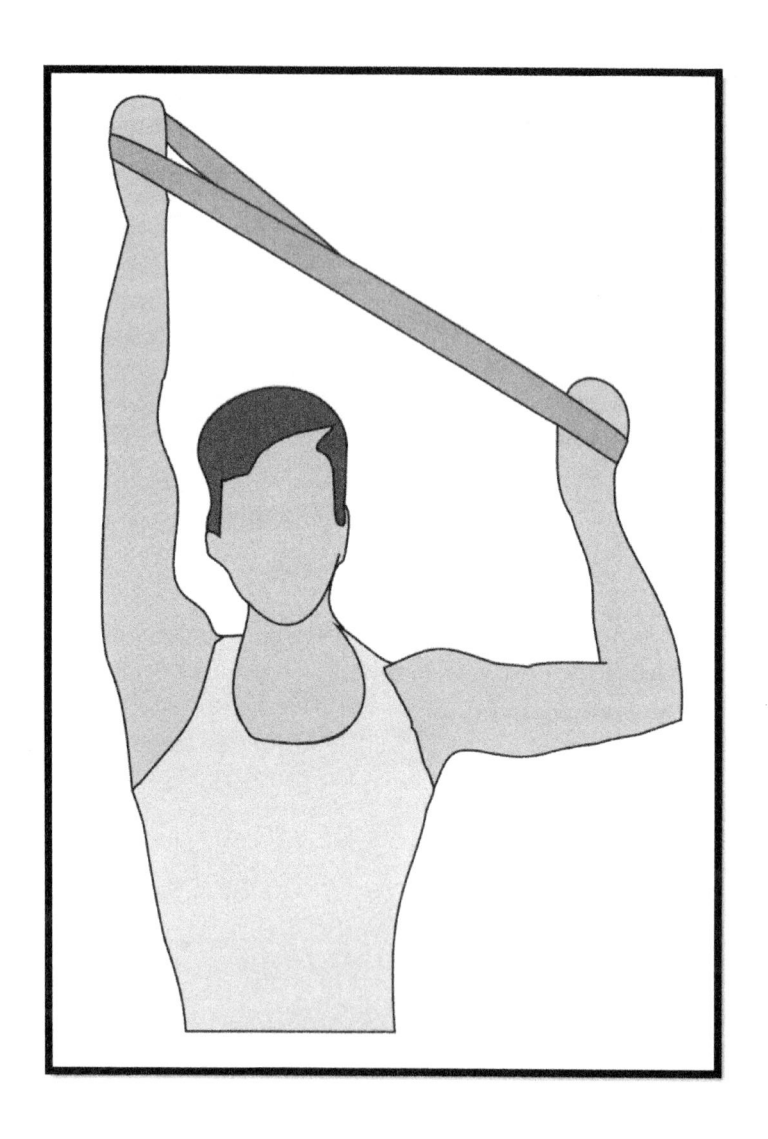

*Effect:* This exercise helps in strengthening of arm and shoulder muscles.

*Difficulty Level:* Advanced

*Start Position:* Hold the resistance loop band in down grip, with arms stretched overhead. Stand tall with your feet hip width distance apart.

*Steps:*

1. Keeping the right arm stretched up, start pulling the band laterally out and down with your left hand, engaging your back muscles.
2. Hold the stretched position for 5 counts and return slowly to the start position.
3. Perform required number of repetitions.
4. Repeat on the other side.

*Fine Tips:*

1. Keep your upper back muscles engaged by pulling down the shoulders down as u do the movement.
2. Your core should be engaged and back tall throughout the movement.

# Dr. Monika Chopra's Fitness Sutra

## Press to Pull

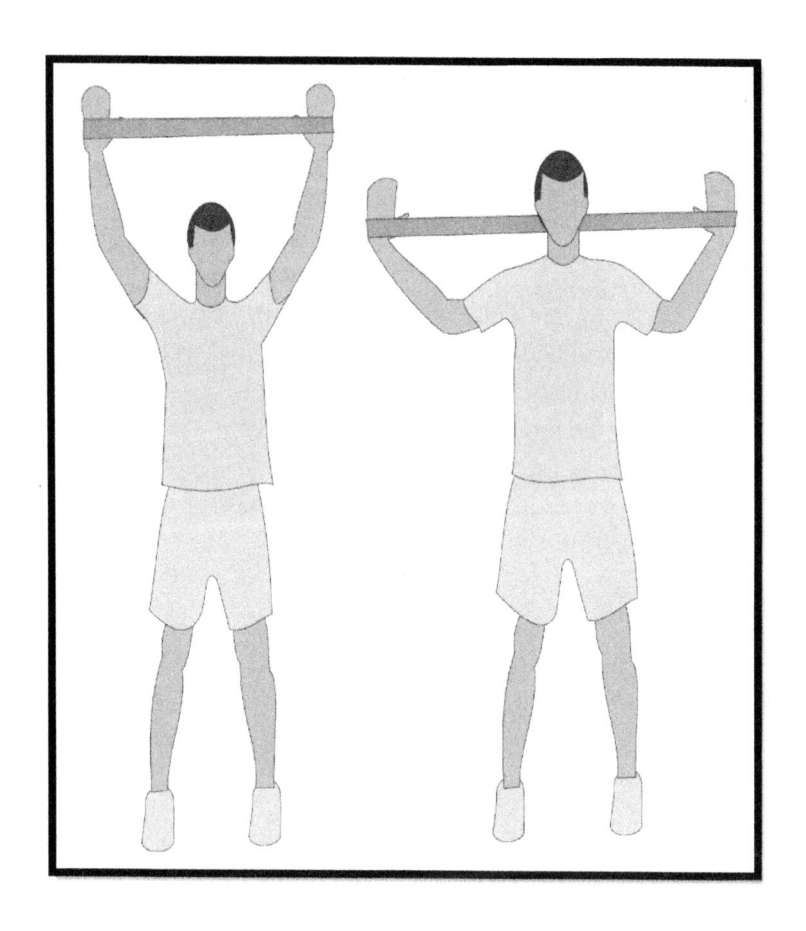

# Exercises with Resistance Loop Bands (2nd Edition)

*Effect:* This exercise helps in strengthening of upper back, shoulder and arm muscles.

*Difficulty Level:* Advanced

*Start Position:* Grasp the loop band in your hands with the hands facing forward, stand tall with core engaged and feet hip width distance apart. Shoulder press overhead the arms keeping tension in the loop.

*Steps:*

1. Maintaining tension in the loop band, take it up and over the head and pull the band down behind the back.
2. Then again maintaining tension in the band, take the band up and overhead getting it down in front of the chest.
3. Repeat this required number of times.

*Fine Tips:*

1. Keep your upper back muscles engaged by pulling down the shoulders as you do the movement.
2. Your core should be engaged and back tall throughout the movement.

# Dr. Monika Chopra's Fitness Sutra

## Shoulder Retraction

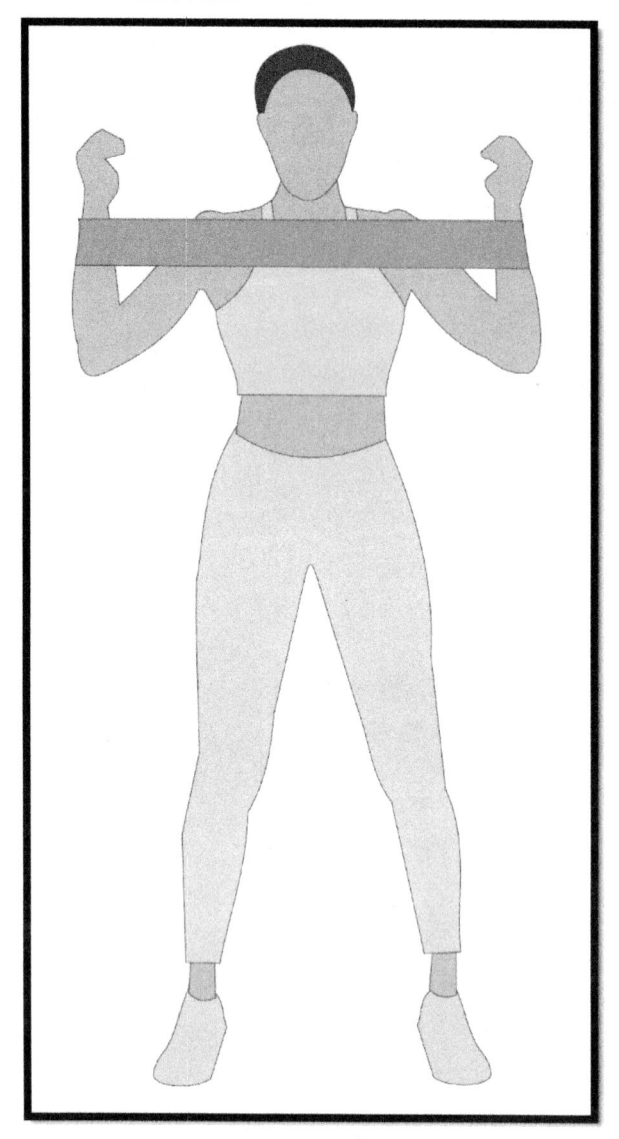

# Exercises with Resistance Loop Bands (2nd Edition)

*Effect:* This exercise helps in strengthening of the shoulder retractor muscles.

*Difficulty Level:* Advanced

*Start Position:* Wrap the resistance loop band around your wrists and raise your arm in a W. Stand tall with core engaged, knees soft and feet grounded.

*Steps:*

1. Retract your shoulder blades, taking the arms behind, as you stretch the loop band slowly.
2. Hold for 5 counts.
3. Return to the start position slowly.
4. Repeat required number of times.

*Fine Tips:*

1. Keep your upper back muscles engaged by pulling down the shoulders as you do the movement.
2. Your core should be engaged and back tall throughout the movement.

# Single Arm Rowing

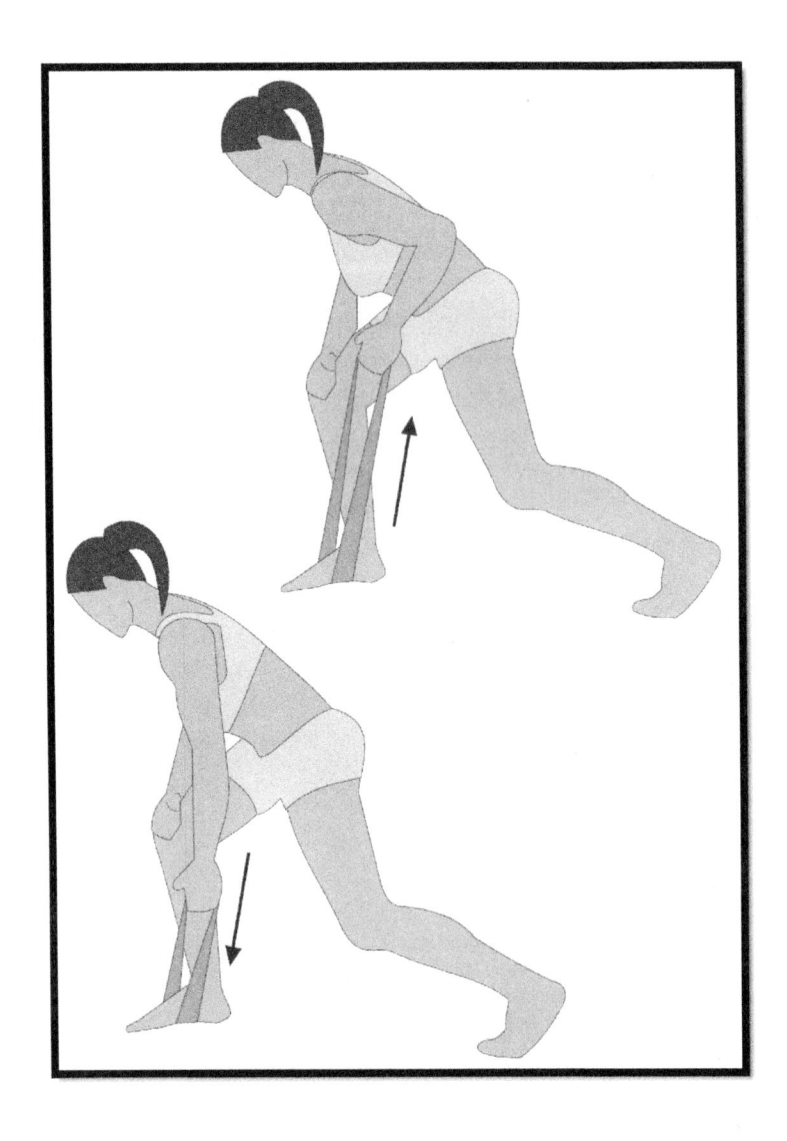

# Exercises with Resistance Loop Bands (2nd Edition)

*Effect:* This exercise helps in strengthening of shoulder extensors and elbow flexors.

*Difficulty Level:* Advanced

*Start Position:* Stand in step standing position with right leg in front. Bend over right leg and rest your right forearm over right thigh, supporting your body. Put the loop band around the right foot and hold its other end with the left hand (hand facing in).

*Steps:*

1. Pull the left hand straight up, bending at the elbow.
2. Hold for 5 counts.
3. Slowly return the hand back to the start position.
4. Do the required number of repetitions.
5. Repeat on the other side.

*Fine Tips:*

1. Keep your trunk stable in the start position as you move the arm.

*"Take care of your body. It's the only place you have to live."*

*— Jim Rohn*

# CHAPTER 7

## Abdominal Exercises

## Oblique Overhead Extension

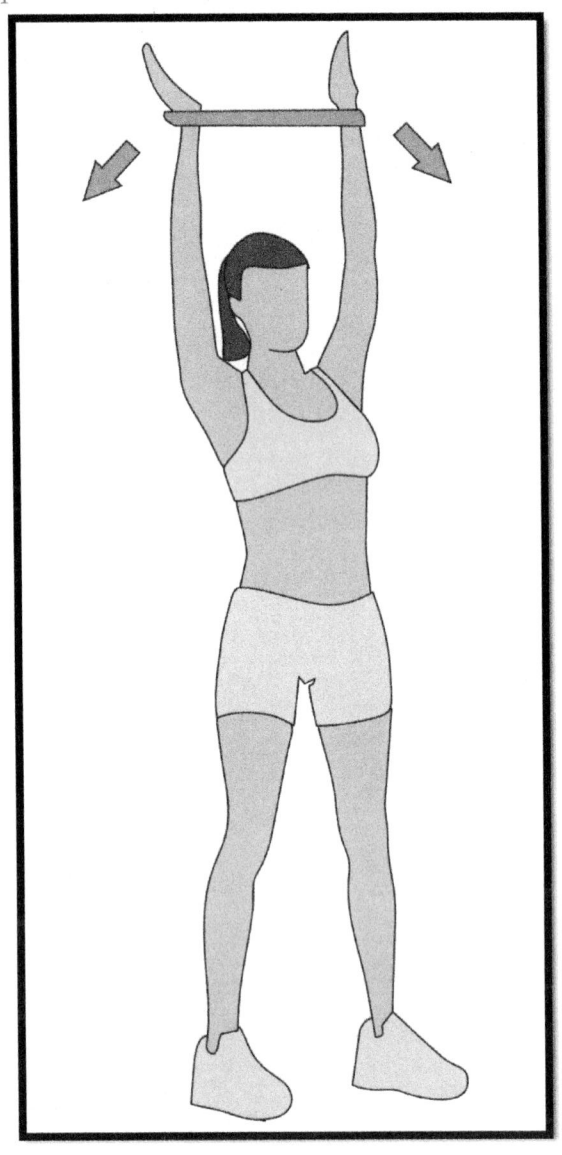

*Effect:* This exercise helps in strengthening of side trunk and abdominal oblique muscles.

*Difficulty Level:* Advanced

*Start Position:* Stand tall with your feet shoulder feet apart and knees slightly bent. Stretch the arms overhead and hold the loop band in the open grip in your hands. Stretch the band out to keep it taut throughout the exercise.

*Steps:*

1. Bend to your right in a controlled manner and feel the stretch in your left obliques.
2. Hold it for 5 counts. Return to the start position.
3. Repeat on the other side.
4. Perform required number of bends.

*Fine Tips:*

1. Keep your back tall, shoulder and core engaged throughout the movement.

## Bicycles

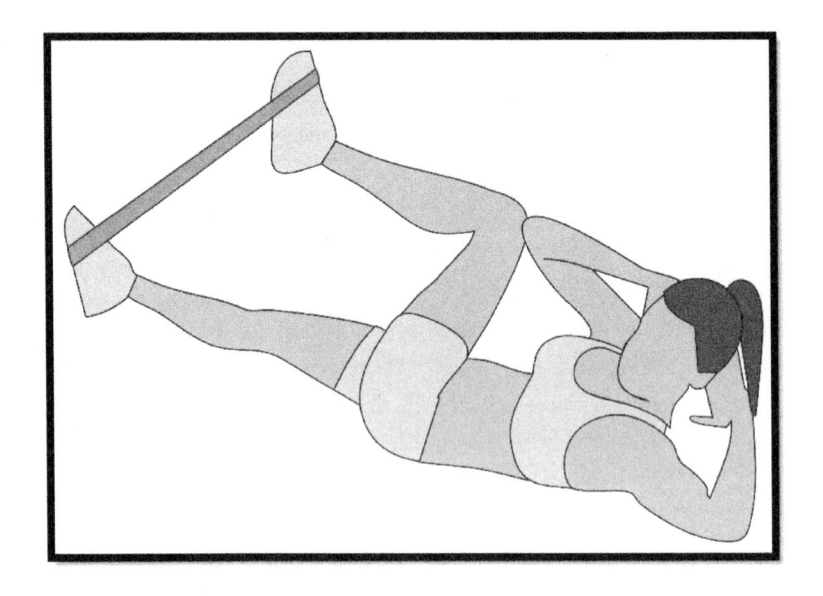

*Effect:* This exercise helps in strengthening of core and lower body muscles.

*Difficulty Level:* Advanced

*Start Position:* Loop the resistance band around your feet and lie down on your back. Place your hands behind your head.

*Steps:*

1. Imprint your back and raise both of your feet about one foot into the air. Pull your left knee towards the abdomen and get your right elbow towards the left knee in a crunching motion. Feel the contraction in your obliques as your elbow touches the knee.
2. Slowly return to the start position
3. Repeat on the other side.

*Fine Tips:*

1. Keep your neck and shoulders relaxed during the exercise.
2. Keep your core engaged throughout the movement.

# Dr. Monika Chopra's Fitness Sutra

## Abdominal Crunch with Rotations

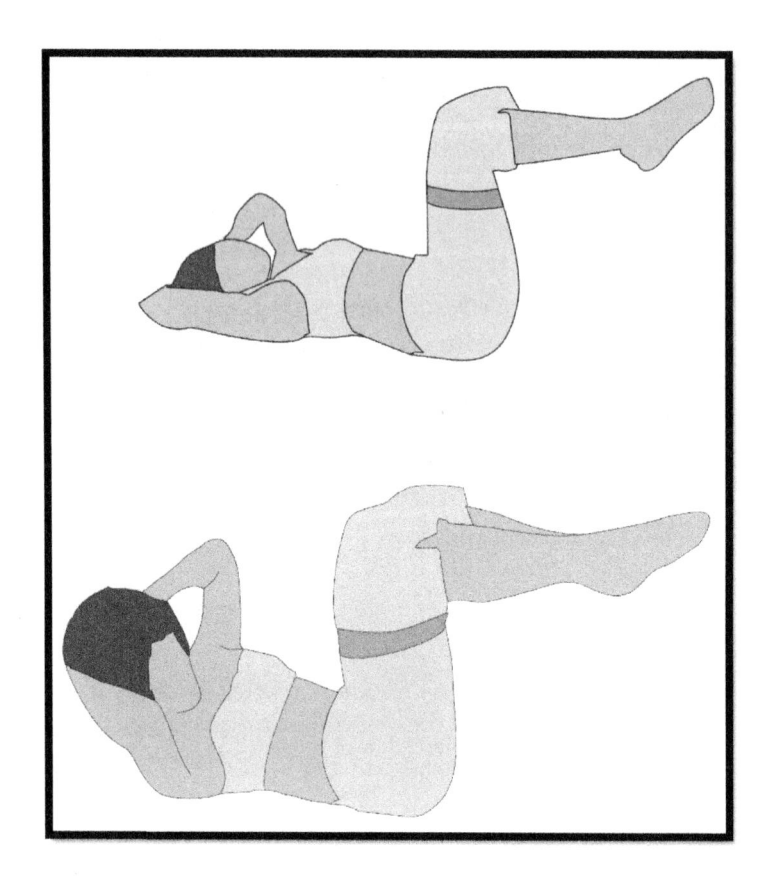

# Exercises with Resistance Loop Bands (2nd Edition)

*Effect:* This exercise helps in strengthening of abdomen oblique muscles.

*Difficulty Level:* Advanced

*Start Position:* Lie down flat on your back with your legs bent to 90 degrees at hip and knees and your lower leg parallel to the floor. Put the loop band around mid-thigh and spread your legs little apart to make the band taut.

*Steps:*

1. Place your hands with fingers interlocked, behind your head. Exhale and raise your back up, bringing your left elbow towards the right knee, crunching the abdomen.
2. Inhale and return to the start position.
3. Repeat on the other side.
4. Perform required number of repetitions.

*Fine Tips:*

1. Keep your neck and shoulders relaxed during the exercise.
2. Keep your core engaged throughout the movement.
3. Keep the band taut throughout the exercise.

## Reverse Crunch

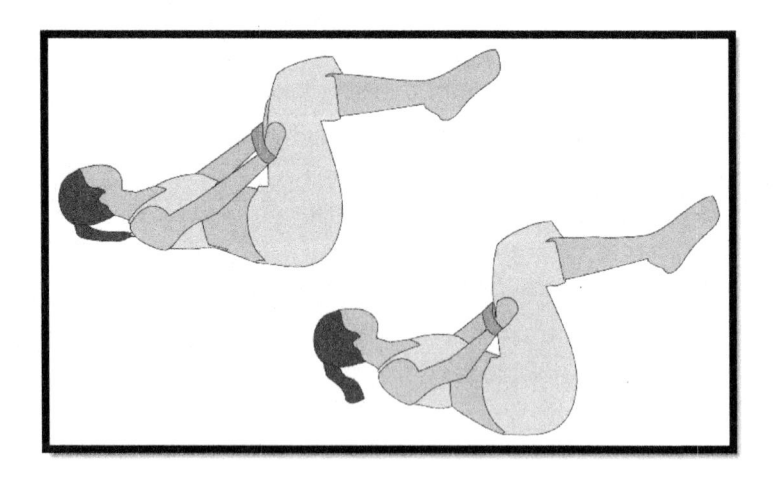

# Exercises with Resistance Loop Bands (2nd Edition)

*Effect:* This exercise helps in strengthening of abdominal muscles.

*Difficulty Level:* Advanced

*Start Position:* Lie down on your back with your legs bent at 90 degrees at hip and knees. Hold the resistance band in down grip against the thigh, with your arms by the side of your body.

*Steps:*

1. Imprint your back contracting your abdominals, roll your hips up, taking your knees towards the face as you raise your upper body slightly above the ground. With each crunch press your hands towards the feet, pushing the resistance of the band against the thigh.
2. Slowly return to the start position.
3. Perform required number of repetitions.

*Fine Tips:*

1. Keep your neck and shoulders relaxed and don't lock your elbows during the exercise.
2. Keep your core engaged throughout the movement.

# CHAPTER 8

## Cool-Down Exercises

# Exercises with Resistance Loop Bands (2nd Edition)

Cool down exercises should always be performed after intensive workout to bring the body back to its normal state. Full body stretches are good cool down exercises. The body is in a very compliant state after exercises. Thus the stretches performed at this time also help to increase the flexibility of the body.

Cool down stretch guidelines
1. Move into the stretched position (where you can feel slight tension) slowly.
2. Inhale and exhale deeply and slowly and let the stretching muscle relax.
3. Hold the stretch for 15 seconds and then slowly return to start position.
4. Perform each stretch twice.

Some stretches which are very beneficial for the body are as follows:

Upper Body Stretch
1. Triceps Stretch (Forward Arm Stretch):

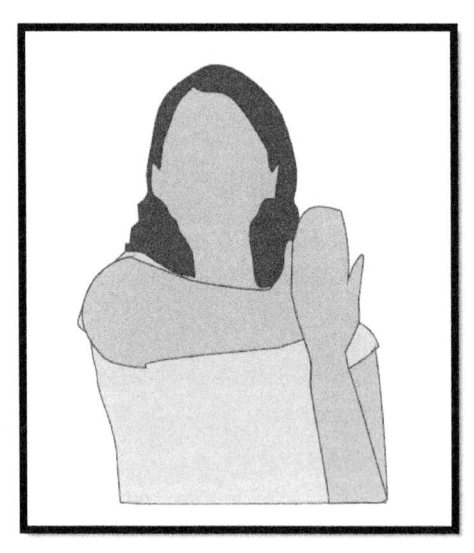

Major muscles worked - rhomboids, deltoids and triceps brachii.
Stand tall with your shoulders levelled and facing forwards and feet hip width distance apart. Extend your right arm to the side at shoulder level with palm facing forward. Move the arm forward and take it across the chest as if to wrap your chest with your arm. Bring the right hand around your left shoulder blade walking your fingertips towards your upper spine to the extent it is comfortable. Feel the stretch on the outside of your right arm, right shoulder and upper back. Breathe deeply into the thoracic spine and upper back, trying to release the stretching muscles. To increase the stretch you may give a slight push at the elbow of the wrapped arm, pulling it towards your chest. Relax. Repeat the above procedure for the left side.

# Exercises with Resistance Loop Bands (2nd Edition)

2. <u>Pectoral Stretch (Backward Arm Stretch)</u>:

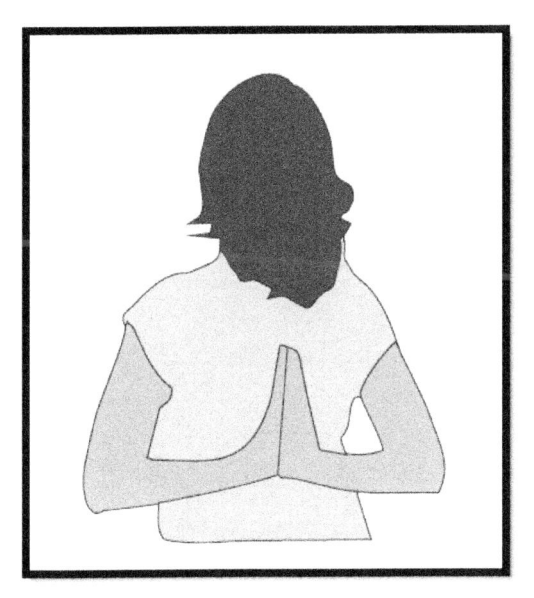

Major muscles worked - pectoralis major and deltoids. Stand tall with your shoulders levelled and facing forward and feet hip width distance apart. Extend your arms to the sides making a "T". Bend your arms at the elbows and bring both hands behind your back till the tip of middle fingers touch each other with little fingers of both hands pressing against the back. Start pushing the middle fingers up slowly. Try to bring all the fingers of left hand in contact with fingers of right hand. Slide the fingers up the spine till the stretch is comfortable. Inhale deeply while stretching the muscles of shoulder, chest, arms and fingers, relaxing them.

3. **Latissimus Dorsi And Triceps Stretch (Upward Arm Stretch):**

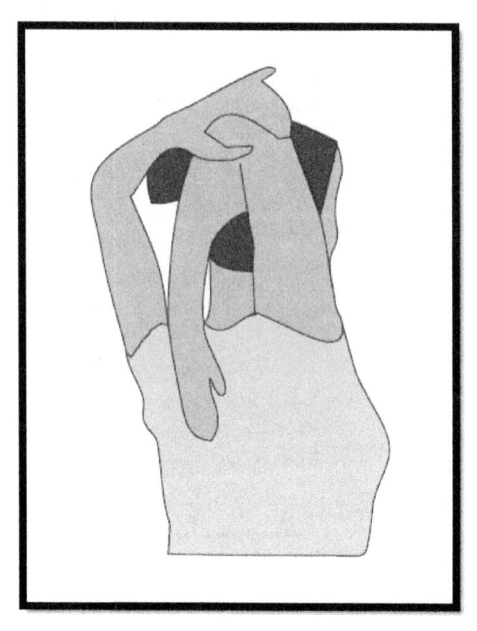

Major muscles worked - Latissimus dorsi and Triceps brachii

Extend your right arm to the side with palm facing up. Raise the arm towards the ceiling and then bend at the elbow till your fingertips reach the spine between your shoulder blades. Walk your fingertips down the spine. Feel the stretch on the outer side of your right arm, upper back and the right side of your trunk. Hold this position and breathe deeply trying to release the stretching muscles of the upper back and around the spine. Come to the start position. Repeat the above procedure for the left side.

# Exercises with Resistance Loop Bands (2nd Edition)

Lower Body Stretch
1. <u>Figure Of Four Forward Bend:</u>

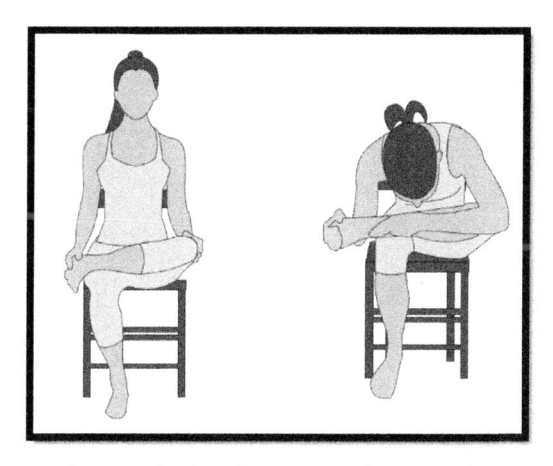

Major muscles worked - gluteus maximus and erector spinae.

Sit tall with feet firmly placed on the ground, hip width distance apart. Place your left ankle over the right knee making a figure of 4 with the legs. Stretch your spine in this position trying to free your hip joint. Let the knee go down under the effect of gravity, opening the left hip joint. Bend forward from this position, leading with your chest while still looking ahead. Breathe while stretching and release the spine and hip joint slowly. Drop your body down towards the floor. Feel the increase in stretch in the hip and spine region. Hold this position. To come out of the above position, raise your spine up, keeping it straight while still keeping the neck and shoulders relaxed. Keep pushing through the right foot into the ground to maintain balance. As the spine comes in an upright position, raise the head and look in front. Come to the start position. Repeat on the other side.

2. <u>Thigh Stretch (Quadriceps Stretch)</u>:

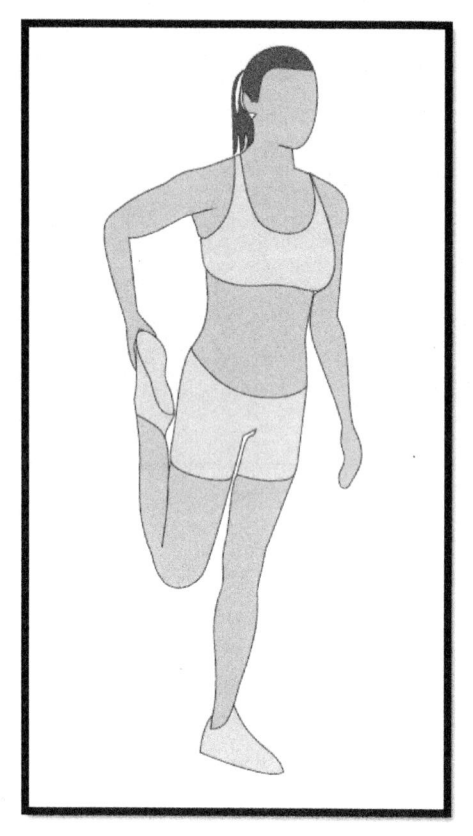

Stand tall with your abdomen tucked in and feet hip width distance apart. Hold a wall or stationary object for balance, Grasp your left foot with your left hand and pull so that your left heel moves towards your left buttock (maintain proper alignment to avoid stress on your knee). You should feel the stretch along the front of your left thigh. Repeat on the other leg.

3. <u>Hamstring Stretch:</u>

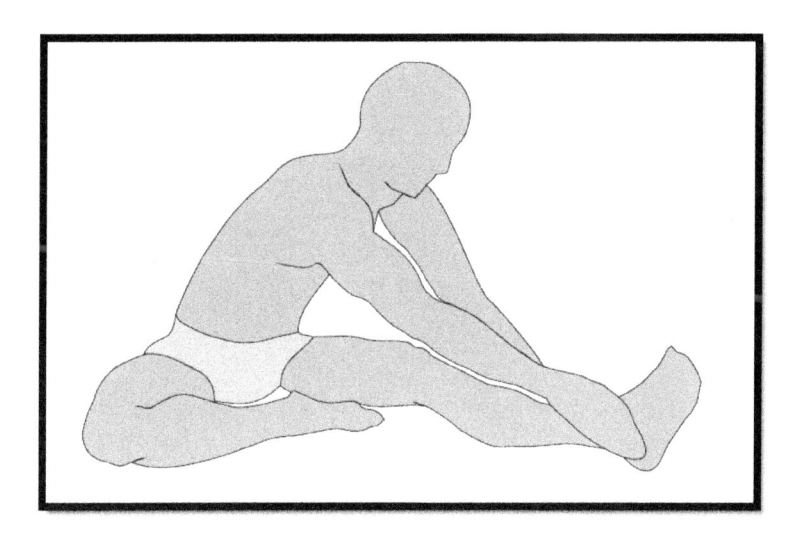

Major muscles worked - Hamstrings and erector spinae. Sit tall in a long sitting position on the floor with your legs hip width distance apart and stretched in front of you. Bend your right leg and place the sole of right foot against the inner side of left thigh, above the knee. Keep your shoulders and hips squared (facing forward). Bend forward at your hips (keeping your back straight and leading with the heart) and move your torso towards your left knee. Be sure to keep your left leg in neutral position with your left toes pointing up. Feel the stretch in your back and hamstring muscles. Switch the leg and repeat on the other side keeping your right leg stretched in front of you.

4. Calf Muscle Stretch:

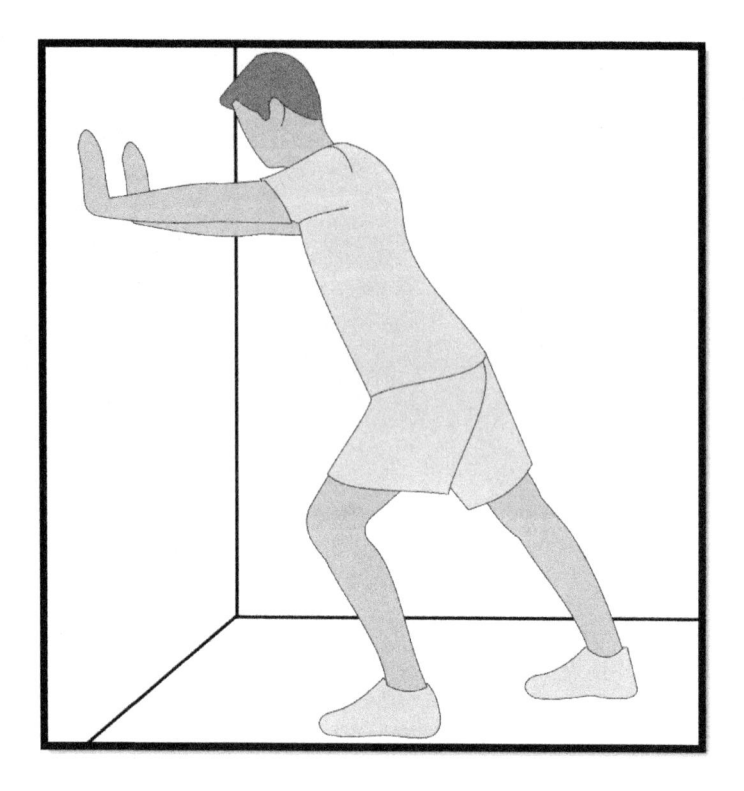

Major muscles involved: Soleus and gastrocnemius.
Stand with your right foot flat on the floor about 1 foot away from the wall (right leg bent) and the left leg stretched straight behind with left heel touching the floor. Place your hands on the wall and bend forwards, keeping your back straight. Feel the stretch behind your left leg. Repeat on the other side.

# CHAPTER 9

Importance of Diet

## Dr. Monika Chopra's Fitness Sutra

Importance of proper diet in your journey to strength & fitness cannot be overstated. Especially for people trying to lose weight, as much as 70% of the fat loss is influenced by dietary choices. This chapter will give you simple tips on what to eat as balanced diet to maintain a lean but strong physique.

1. Eat protein with each meal – adequate amount of protein consumption is essential for muscle tissue recovery during strength training program. Whole proteins should be part of each of your meals. Proteins keep you full for longer time thus helping in fat loss. Protein rich foods have a higher thermic effect, thus more of the meal is burned during digestion. Each day, one should eat 1g of protein for every 1 pound of body weight.

2. Eat vegetables with each meal – vegetables are fibre rich and thus fill you up with less carbs intake. Fibre also improves digestion. Vegetables contain many valuable vitamins, phytochemicals, and antioxidants for better health. You should aim to eat at least half a plate of veggies at each meal. Vegetables contain lots of fibre that would help in your bowel movements that may otherwise get adversely affected with a high protein diet.

3. Limit your carbohydrate intake – carbohydrates are high calorie food. If you are doing strength training to reduce body fat you should limit your carbohydrate intake thus limiting calorie intake.

4. <u>Avoid processed food</u> – avoid processed food and try to consume food mostly in natural state. Processed foods (generally all the eatables that are made in factories like soda, cookies, cereals (including bars), frozen food etc.) are invariably high in sugar & salt. Sugar can be disguised as other ingredients like HFCS (i.e. High Fructose Corn Syrup). Factories put in high amounts of sugar & fats to compensate for the loss of taste that invariably occurs due to mass production & packaging.

5. <u>Eat good fats</u> – fats do not necessarily make you fat. Considerate amount of fat is actually required while strength training. Fats keep you full for longer periods of time and provide essential fatty acids. Include some nuts & dry fruits in your meal plan for snack times.

6. <u>Drink lots of water</u> – It is essential to keep yourself hydrated all the time; especially during workouts as you tend to lose a lot of water through sweating. Dehydration from lack of drinking may cause headaches for some folks. Also you need water for proper muscle recovery. Do not go by any thumb rules for water intake - just ensure to drink as & when you feel thirsty. If you do not feel the need to empty your bladder every few hours, then it's a sign that you are not taking in enough water to flush all the toxins.

# CHAPTER 10

## Training Regimes

# Exercises with Resistance Loop Bands (2nd Edition)

## *Beginners' Regime*

In 1st week, do 1 set of 15 repetitions each.
In 2nd week, do 2 sets of 15 repetitions each.
In the 3rd & 4th weeks, do 3 sets of 15 repetitions each.

Repeat the Beginners' regime for 4 weeks. Increase the resistance level of the band, when you are comfortable with one resistance level.

Day 1 & Day 5

Upper Body Exercises
- Front Triceps Extension
- Horizontal Arm Extension
- Vertical Arm Extension
- Bicep Curl
- Internal Rotation
- External Rotation
- Hand Scrunches
- Seated Concentration Curl
- Wrist Curl

Abdominal Exercise
- Oblique Overhead Extension

Day 3 & Day 7

Lower Body Exercises
- Lying Leg Raise
- Standing Hip Abduction
- Leg Extension
- Supinated Clamshell
- Thigh Thrust
- Lateral Walk
- Backwards Leg Swing
- Standing Hip Adduction
- Standing Hip Extension
- Seated Hip Abduction
- Ankle Internal Rotation

# Exercises with Resistance Loop Bands (2nd Edition)

## *Advanced Regime*

In 1st week, do 2 sets of 15 repetitions each.
In 2nd week, do 3 sets of 15 repetitions each.
3rd week onwards, do 3 sets of 20 repetitions each.

Increase the resistance level of the band, when you are comfortable with one resistance level.

Day 1 & Day 5

Upper Body Exercises
- Rear Triceps Extension
- Rear Arm Extension
- Lateral Arm Raise (Rotator Cuff)

Chest & Back Exercises
- Lateral Push Up
- Lateral Pull Down
- Press to Pull
- Shoulder Retraction
- Single Arm Rowing

Abdominal Exercises
- Bicycles
- Abdominal Crunch with Rotations

Day 3 & Day 7

Lower Body Exercises
- Bridge Thrust
- One Leg Hip Thrust
- Side Step Squats
- Lying Hip Abduction
- Band Squats
- Clam Shell
- Standing Hip Flexion
- Single Leg Loop Bridge
- Seated Leg Extension

Abdominal Exercise
- Reverse Crunch

Full Body Exercise
- Bear Crawls

Exercises with Resistance Loop Bands (2nd Edition)

## Bonus

I hope you liked the book and have already started doing these exercises. Please give me a review on Amazon

https://www.fitness-sutra.com/go?id=121279

SCAN ME!

I have created easy to use quick reference charts of the regimes (beginners / advanced) suggested in the previous chapter of this book. These can be downloaded as ready printable files from

https://www.fitness-sutra.com/go?id=121151

SCAN ME!

You can also subscribe to my mailing list to get more tips & motivation to do these exercises. I try to keep my subscribers abreast of the latest developments in the field of strength training.

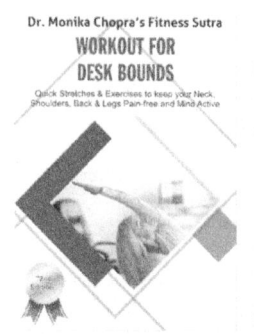

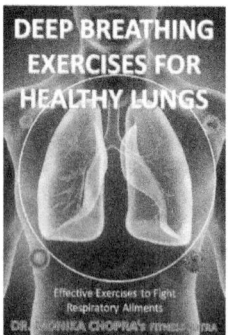

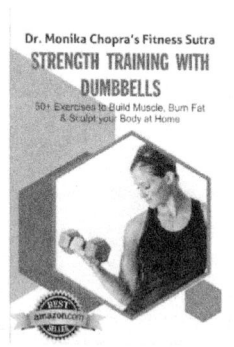

## More Books by Dr. Monika Chopra

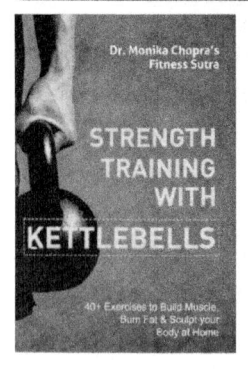

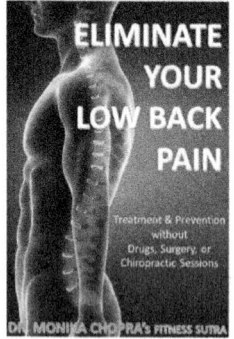

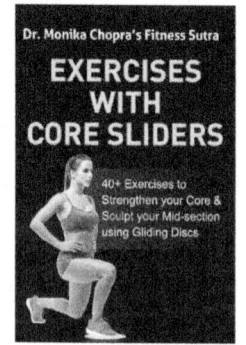

https://www.fitness-sutra.com/go?id=122514

Printed in Great Britain
by Amazon